ANESTHESIA AND THE CLASSICS

FRONT COVER ILLUSTRATION: The lyre is an ancient string instrument (variously numbered strings, most commonly 4, 7 or 10) said to have been invented by Hermes, the messenger of the gods. It was used to provide musical accompaniment during the delivery of lyrical ("singing") poetry. Eventually and metaphorically, the poet became the lyre, an honorific to his skill and articulation. This illustration of a Muse (Kalliope) playing the lyre also shows an inscription on the rock upon which she is seated: *Helikon* (Ηελικου). *Helikon* was a Boiotian (central Greece) mountain god who, as a god, was a direct competitor in musical contests judged by the Muses, and as a mountain, was the site of such lyrical competitions involving the Muses and judged by Hermes. As an adjective, *helikos* represents the dialectic of size – how great and how small, and figuratively, the process of becoming great or "coming of age." (Staatliche Antikensammlungen, public domain, via Wikimedia Commons)

ANESTHESIA AND THE CLASSICS

Essays on avatars of professional values

Robert S. Holzman
M.D., M.A. (Hon), FAAP
Senior Associate in Perioperative
Anesthesia, Boston Children's Hospital
Professor of Anaesthesia, Harvard
Medical School, Boston, MA

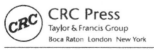

CRC Press is an imprint of the
Taylor & Francis Group, an **informa** business

First edition published 2022
by CRC Press
6000 Broken Sound Parkway NW, Suite 300, Boca Raton, FL 33487-2742

and by CRC Press
2 Park Square, Milton Park, Abingdon, Oxon, OX14 4RN

© 2022 Taylor & Francis Group, LLC

CRC Press is an imprint of Taylor & Francis Group, LLC

This book contains information obtained from authentic and highly regarded sources. While all reasonable efforts have been made to publish reliable data and information, neither the author[s] nor the publisher can accept any legal responsibility or liability for any errors or omissions that may be made. The publishers wish to make clear that any views or opinions expressed in this book by individual editors, authors or contributors are personal to them and do not necessarily reflect the views/opinions of the publishers. The information or guidance contained in this book is intended for use by medical, scientific or health-care professionals and is provided strictly as a supplement to the medical or other professional's own judgement, their knowledge of the patient's medical history, relevant manufacturer's instructions and the appropriate best practice guidelines. Because of the rapid advances in medical science, any information or advice on dosages, procedures or diagnoses should be independently verified. The reader is strongly urged to consult the relevant national drug formulary and the drug companies' and device or material manufacturers' printed instructions, and their websites, before administering or utilizing any of the drugs, devices or materials mentioned in this book. This book does not indicate whether a particular treatment is appropriate or suitable for a particular individual. Ultimately it is the sole responsibility of the medical professional to make his or her own professional judgements, so as to advise and treat patients appropriately. The authors and publishers have also attempted to trace the copyright holders of all material reproduced in this publication and apologize to copyright holders if permission to publish in this form has not been obtained. If any copyright material has not been acknowledged please write and let us know so we may rectify in any future reprint.

Except as permitted under U.S. Copyright Law, no part of this book may be reprinted, reproduced, transmitted, or utilized in any form by any electronic, mechanical, or other means, now known or hereafter invented, including photocopying, microfilming, and recording, or in any information storage or retrieval system, without written permission from the publishers.

For permission to photocopy or use material electronically from this work, access www.copyright.com or contact the Copyright Clearance Center, Inc. (CCC), 222 Rosewood Drive, Danvers, MA 01923, 978-750-8400. For works that are not available on CCC please contact mpkbookspermissions@tandf.co.uk

Trademark notice: Product or corporate names may be trademarks or registered trademarks and are used only for identification and explanation without intent to infringe.

Library of Congress Cataloging-in-Publication Data
Names: Holzman, Robert S., 1951– author.
Title: Anesthesia and the classics: essays on avatars of professional values/Robert S. Holzman.
Description: First edition. | Boca Raton: CRC Press, 2022. |
Includes bibliographical references and index.
Identifiers: LCCN 2021032166 (print) | LCCN 2021032167 (ebook) |
ISBN 9781032049014 (paperback) | ISBN 9781032062419 (hardback) |
ISBN 9781003201328 (ebook)
Subjects: MESH: Anesthesiology | Professionalism | Virtues |
Interprofessional Relations | Greek World | Essay
Classification: LCC RD81 (print) | LCC RD81 (ebook) |
NLM WO 209 | DDC 617.9/6–dc23
LC record available at https://lccn.loc.gov/2021032166
LC ebook record available at https://lccn.loc.gov/2021032167

ISBN: 978-1-03-206241-9 (hbk)
ISBN: 978-1-03-204901-4 (pbk)
ISBN: 978-1-00-320132-8 (ebk)

DOI: 10.1201/9781003201328

Typeset in New Baskerville Std
by Newgen Publishing UK

CONTENTS

Preface ix

Introduction: Looking Backward, Looking Forward: The Legacy of Janus   1

Part I The Human Condition   7

1 Disease: The *Nosoi*   9

2 Health and Healing: The *Asklepiades*   17

3 Uncertainty: *Nyx* and Her Children   29

4 Safety: *Soteria*   41

5 The Spirits of Pain and Suffering: The *Algea*   49

6 Anesthesia: "A Not-Feeling Pain"   55

Part II Qualities   67

7 Scholarship: *Kheiron*   71

8 Skill: *Tekhne*   83

9 Beauty and Grace: *Kalleis*, *Aphrodite* and *Apollo*   91

10 Wisdom: *Sophia*   101

Part III The Emotions — 111

11 Strife and Harmony: *Eris* and *Harmonia* — 113

12 Fear and Panic: *Phobos* — 121

13 Love: The *Erotes* — 129

Part IV Morality — 143

14 Truth and Lies: *Aletheia* and *Pseudologos* — 145

15 Respect: *Aidos* — 155

16 Justice: *Dike* — 163

17 Kindliness: *Philoprosyne* — 171

18 Self-Control: *Sophrosyne* — 181

Part V Voice — 189

19 Consolation: *Paregoros* — 191

20 Eloquence: *Kalliope* — 199

Part VI Actions — 209

21 Effort and Laziness: *Hormes* and *Aergia* — 211

22 Victory and Retreat: *Nike* and *Palioxis* — 217

Part VII Society   227

23 Law and Order/Lawlessness, Disorder
    and Ruin: *Nomos* and *Eunomia/Dysnomia*
    and *Ate*   231

24 Justice and Democracy: *Dike* and *Demokratia*   241

    Postface   251
    Index   255

PREFACE

The operating room is a crucible for professionalism and a laboratory for professional development. It requires expertise in anatomy, physiology and pharmacology, balancing of certainty and uncertainty, tolerance for and an understanding of patients' self-control and its abandonment, crucial and rapid decision-making and leadership, and the calculus of democratic input balanced with individual authority, power and responsibility. It is about relationships not only between individuals but also relationships of time, space and self-development – professionalism.

As words go, "profession" has been around a relatively long time (13th century, as a religious term for one who "professes" a belief or faith, and publicly professes such by declaration, or oath). This verb became nounified when its use broadened to the calling that one professed. The learned professions (those that required specialized knowledge, long, rigorous academic preparation and an oath) were recognized as medicine, the law and religion.* *Professionalism*, the requisite qualities for practicing a profession, appeared in the mid-19th century, with astonishingly increased usage.

No longer limited to the learned professions, "professionalism" has been broadly deployed to describe cognitive, technical and judgmental competence, behaviors ranging from communication skills to civility and wisdom, typically within the

---

* Historically, the practices of law, medicine and theology, requiring advanced knowledge:

> *after a prolonged course of specialized instruction and study. The first requirement is that the knowledge be of an advanced type. Second, it must be knowledge in a field of science or learning, distinguishing the professions from the mechanical arts. Historically, there was also a requirement for literacy.*

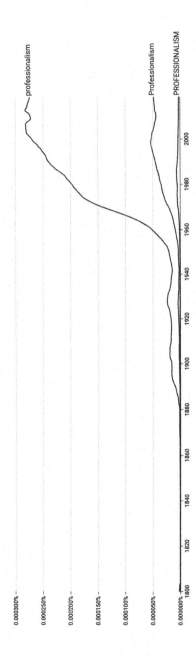

confines of a particular occupation but not limited to the learned professions – for example, a professional athlete.

Medicine as a profession carries some specific obligations. There is a context within which the above behaviors will be conveyed to colleagues, students and patients. Moreover, a substantial amount of professional growth should come from reflection about one's experiences caring for real patients – an appreciation of **the human condition**.

Those conditions span patients who are healthy and ill and place specific demands on the provider such as empathy, knowledge, generosity, and respect, a "family" of values that was personified by the Ancients in the *family of Asklepios*. The healers, as well as those being healed, remained *uncertain* about their fate, represented by Night and her children. Wanting *Safety*, patients also long for the daring and boldness that may be required for the restoration of their health. *Pain* is likely to accompany their suffering and uncertainty, relieved by the miracle of a "not-feeling pain:" – "*Anesthesia*."

What **qualities** does it take to be a professional? Certainly *scholarship*, as embodied by *Kheiron* the Centaur, teacher of *Akhilles* and the first medical educator. In addition to Scholarship, *skill* is required, represented by *Tekhne*, the spirit of art, technical skill and craft, inseparable from *Hephaistos* (Vulcan) and the *Muses*. Moving beyond competencies into the realm of milestones and entrustable professional activities, something more is required – independent mastery of beauty and articulation in craft and in thought that are integral to the highest standards of practice, across all specialties. *Beauty* and *Grace* embody the highest technical performance levels for any specialty and include the ability to be articulate with colleagues and patients in the spoken and written word. Even these lofty achievements are the penultimate step. The ultimate step, *wisdom*, personified by *Sophia*, crowns the previous values as an essential quality of mature professionalism.

What of the **emotional** milieu of medical professionals and their human relationships? Until relatively recently, medical care was rendered not in collaboration but rather solitarily, and with intransigent pride. The stunning explosion of medical information and discovery as well as a deeper understanding of the complexities of medical illness, cast against a background of increasing survival of progressively complex patients compels us to collaborate – live "in *Harmony*" – with our colleagues. In the operating room melting pot, the tension between *harmony* and *strife* has existed since the positioning of surgeon and anesthetist north and south of the ether screen, occasionally referred to as the "blood-brain barrier." At times, *fear*, and every so often, *panic*, will enter the emotional milieu as inevitabilities of uncertainty. However, *love*, in its numerous manifestations – love of scholarship, craft, camaraderie, and patient care – must conquer all, in order to truly energize and engage the professional. The closing line in a talk given by Dr. Francis W. Peabody to the students at Harvard Medical School on October 21, 1926 – "the secret of the care of the patient is in *caring* for the patient,"[1] speaks to this ideal.

Morality[†] influences interpersonal relationships in every interaction, and so it is with medicine and the care of our fellow human beings. At the personal level this involves the provider–patient relationship while on a macro-level morality influences interprofessional and intergroup cooperation. Collaboration in groups and teamwork is now recognized as vital to the rapid and effective implementation of the explosion in medical knowledge. Civility between "team" members (even if they don't regard themselves as a formal team) is essential to effective communication. Here, the spirits of Classical morality illustrate the salient issues. *Truth (Aletheia), Respect (Aedos), Justice (Dike), Kindliness (Philophrosyne)* and *Self-Control (Sophrosyne)* are key components of professional relationships, with patients as well as colleagues. The avoidance of *Laziness (Aergia)* underscores the commitment to sincere effort that professionals must exercise.

The cultivation of one's professional *voice* is not specifically identified as a goal within typical lists of professional qualities, yet it is crucial to interpersonal-professional relationships with patients, essential to accurate communication with colleagues and collaborators and critical to the advancement of scientific inquiry and reporting. Articulation has intimate as well as bold aspects. A professional's ability to provide *consolation*, Classically represented by *Paregoros*, is part of empathetic and humanistic medicine. At the same time, articulation, writ large, is essential to collegial collaboration, accuracy of scientific communication

---

[†] From the Latin *moralis* "manner, character, proper behavior."

and critical to teaching, the essential meaning of "doctoring."‡ This broad, and typically more public form of articulation, in both the spoken and written word, is often referred to as *eloquence*, represented by *Kalliope*.

Actions, said to speak louder than words, operationalize one's public and private voice. *Hormes* represented effort in the Classics, while the dialectic of Victory and Retreat was the domain of *Nike* and *Palimonies*.

Finally, the role the professional assumes within *society* is governed by explicit and implicit rules – the explicit man-made rules of law (and their disregard – lawlessness) represented by the dialectic of *Nomos* and *Dysnomia*, and the ideals upon which professional advice, care and availability remain – Democracy (*Demokratia*) and Justice (*Dike*).

These values – understanding the human condition, the emotional milieu of medical care, professional morality, the development of one's voice, the commitment to action, and the societal context of the law, justice and democracy – enrich and amplify the more relatively anemic "professionalism" and place an evolving discipline – call it "professionology" – into a more vivid context because of the attachment of values to behaviors.

Even if we can't exactly *define* professionalism and the attempt to parse the measurable behaviors of professionalism into competencies is overly reductionistic, is it nevertheless possible to employ professional development tools to teach professionalism? Stern and Papadakis outlined three essential components of teaching professionalism: setting expectations, providing experiences, and evaluating outcomes.[5] Within the category of providing experiences, they addressed methods of conveying the hidden curriculum[6]§ (including professional values), the role of role models, and the power of parables. Parables – storytelling – take place every day, formally in the lecture hall and even more frequently at the bedside. Books have been written with vignettes that act as medical morality plays for these principles

---

‡ Docere (L) means to instruct, teach, or point out, first used by Cicero in *De Oratore*. (55 BCE).

§ A hidden curriculum is a side effect of an education, "(lessons) which are learned but not openly intended" such as norms, values, and beliefs conveyed in the classroom and the social environment.

and values.[7,8] The attempt to incorporate such informality into a formal curriculum is a challenge, but one for which a storytelling approach such as the relationships between mythology and abstract concepts of professionalism may be a perfect fit.

In my specialty of anesthesiology, involuntary unconsciousness, the core of the anesthetic state, holds a transcendent discomfort for people. As a (professional) purveyor of this state, I have periodically turned back, via allegory, to ancient teachers to look for help with this discomfiting concept, as old as the struggle between self-control and relief from pain and suffering. Unconsciousness, uncertainty and the watershed between sleep, death and dreams are the emotional and cognitive provinces of the anesthesia clinician. This poignancy is captured in the clinician's brief contact with a patient at the threshold of abandonment of emotional as well as physiological security.

There are almost 47,000 anesthesiologists, 44,000 certified registered nurse anesthetists (CRNAs), and more than 1,300 Anesthesia Assistants (AAs) actively practicing in the United States. Thousands more provide healthcare within the milieu of the perioperative state – postanesthesia care unit nurses as well as nurses on the surgical wards, preoperative clinic nursing staff, anesthesia technicians, and various assistants in the operating room, as well as our surgical and many medical colleagues. Anesthetic practice, using the term to include, in broad extension, those non-anesthetists with whom we are closely associated, is founded upon principles of expertise, skill, focus, mindfulness and collaboration, all of which are integral to professionalism.

In an essay in the *AMA Journal of Ethics*, McGoldrick acknowledged that anesthesiology "began as a craft or trade rather than a true profession."[9] This history, as it began and then remained a core characteristic of the clinical practice of anesthesiology, can be ideally placed within the context of *Hephaistos* and *Tekhne*. With time and suitable advancement (through *eloquence*),[3,10–12] the specialty progressed to a level of intellectual achievement equally in keeping with the scholarship of *Kheiron*, the beauty and grace of *Kalleis, Aphrodite* and *Apollo*, while striving for the wisdom of *Sophia*.

For the sake of translating the qualitative aspects of professionalism into quantitative metrics,[11,13] behaviors and competencies must be defined in order to measure inter-rater reliability – Likert scales, and the like – and therefore may not require the same depth of contemplation as a value or trait possessed by or lacking in an individual. Because of the narrowness required to define a behavior, breadth may be sacrificed and compliant behaviors appear to be "prescribed" – rules. However, rules, no matter how well illustrated by vignettes or operational definitions, do not inform the prediction of a broad range of behaviors within a principle in the same way as attaching a persona. When we ponder, "How would Jane do this?" we combine our knowledge of Jane's personality, prior behaviors and choices, value systems, etc. into our answer. Our knowledge of the individual's characteristics (the *persona*) allows us to factor in numerous bits of data, factual, emotional, impressionistic, etc., into the answer. While such answers are tainted by our own values and perceptions eclipsing the "objectivity" of the prediction of Jane's behavior, humans do this all the time. The Greeks knew this well, and often used allegory to promote a nuanced level of understanding and teaching.

At the beginning of the modern history of surgical anesthesia, publicly acknowledged as October 16, 1846 (the first public demonstration at Massachusetts General Hospital of ether's efficacy in providing insensibility to surgical pain), Crawford Long in Georgia and William Clarke in Rochester, New York, had already used ether and nitrous oxide for intentional surgical anesthesia, without publicity, in 1842. Yet the public voice of William T.G. Morton fueled the worldwide recognition of this remarkable achievement, reinforced by the famous phrase of Dr. John Collins Warren in the Ether Dome at Massachusetts General Hospital – "Gentlemen, this is no humbug!" Morton did not hesitate to use his "voice." Neither did Warren.

The principles, values and traits of professionalism and the applicable Classical allegories are by no means specific to the practice of anesthesia; all medical specialties and indeed a wide range of classically learned and other professions and crafts (business, athletics, fine arts) can – and do – subscribe to these principles.

Recognizing this crucial yet imperfectly developed and evolving qualitative area of practice called professionalism has prompted my desire for a more lyrical understanding of the traits required for practice. The avatars that follow, Classical *personae* of essential professional traits, have applicability far beyond clinical anesthesia practice and health care and hopefully provide a richer conversational vocabulary for the ideals of professional development.

RSH

References

1. Peabody F. The care of the patient. *JAMA* 1927; 88: 877–82.
2. Flexner A. *Medical Education in the United States and Canada: A Report to the Carnegie Foundation for the Advancement of Teaching.* New York, NY, The Carnegie Foundation for the Advancement of Teaching, 1910.
3. Greene N. *Anesthesiology and the University.* Philadelphia, Lippincott, 1975.
4. American Board of Internal Medicine Foundation. Medical professionalism in the new millennium: a physician charter. *Ann Intern Med* 2002; 136: 243–6.
5. Stern D, Papadakis M. The developing physician — becoming a professional. *N Engl J Med* 2006; 355: 1794–6.
6. Martin J. What Should We Do with a Hidden Curriculum When We Find One?, *The Hidden Curriculum and Moral Education.* Edited by Giroux H, Purpel D. Berkeley, California, McCutchan Publishing Corporation, 1983, pp 122–1397.
7. Nuland S. *The Soul of Medicine: Tales From the Bedside.* New York, Kaplan Publishing, 2009.
8. Fanning G. *Things I Didn't Learn in Medical School: Tough Lessons from a Lifetime of Practice.* Bloomington, Indiana, Xlibris Corporation, 2012.
9. McGoldrick K. The history of professionalism in anesthesiology. *AMA J Ethics* 2015; 17: 258–64.
10. Chestnut D. On the road to professionalism. *Anesthesiology* 2017; 126: 780–6.
11. Tetzlaff J. Professionalism in anesthesiology: "What is it?" or "I know it when I see it." *Anesthesiology* 2009; 110: 700–2.
12. Vandam L. Early American anesthetists: the origins of professionalism in anesthesia. *Anesthesiology* 1973; 38: 264–74.
13. Dorotta I, Staszak J, Takla A, Tetzlaff J. Teaching and evaluating professionalism for anesthesiology residents. *J Clin Anesth* 2006; 18: 148–60.

INTRODUCTION: LOOKING BACKWARD, LOOKING FORWARD: THE LEGACY OF JANUS

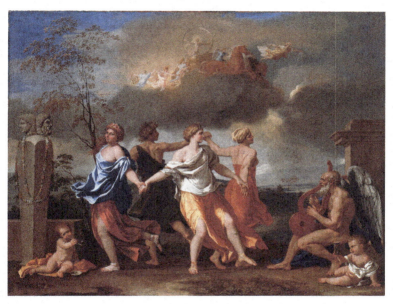

"A Dance to the Music of Time" (1634–1635) by Nicolas Poussin (1594–1665). The four dancing figures originally represented the four seasons, but as Poussin progressed with the painting, his theme changed to the passage of time in the context of the different stages of life and fortune. The four then came to represent *Poverty* (the only male figure, shoeless, darker, and in the background), *Labor* (as well muscled as the male figure, also barefoot, grasping for the hand of …) *Wealth* (with golden sandals and robes, and a disconnected, distant gaze) and *Pleasure* (looking at YOU, the viewer, with a smirk). The passage of time's microcosm, the day, is indicated by the chariot of *Apollo. Aurora*, the goddess of dawn, precedes Apollo's chariot. *Time*, playing a lyre, waits at the end of the cycle, while a statue to

Janus (note the unbearded Janus facing the beginning and the bearded Janus, facing the end) is positioned at the beginning as well as gazing at the end. Everything else in the image is in motion except for the implacable Janus. (Nicolas Poussin, public domain, via Wikimedia Commons.)

An anesthetic has a beginning, middle and end, typically known as induction, maintenance and emergence. Of course, the relationship between anesthetists and patients extends longer than that because one has to meet the patient preoperatively for a history and physical examination as well as an explanation of the anesthetic experience, the risks, benefits and alternatives, and answer any questions or uncertainties. The "pre-induction" time is spent with the patient settling in to the preoperative holding area, changing clothes, having an intravenous line placed, and obtaining baseline vital signs. Typically, at this point the patient, having met the holding area nursing staff, will then meet the operating room nursing staff, the anesthesia team and the surgical team, answer any last-minute questions, have the surgical site examined once again and clearly marked by the surgeon, and often receive some sedation medications to alleviate preoperative anxiety. The patient is then taken to the operating room, physiological monitors are placed such as electrocardiogram leads, a blood pressure cuff and a pulse oximeter to measure oxygen saturation in the blood. These are non-invasive monitors; it is not uncommon to have invasive monitors placed at this time as well, particularly for very sick and marginally stable patients or prior to starting a complex surgical procedure. These invasive monitors often consist of catheters placed in an artery to measure arterial blood pressure directly or in a large vein in the neck with the catheter threaded into various cardiac chambers to measure intracardiac pressures. Medications are administered ("**induction** medications") and typically an endotracheal tube is placed into the patient's trachea to provide gas exchange and mechanical ventilation during surgery. Patients are kept asleep with varying combinations of intravenous medications as well as potent inhalation anesthetics in a careful balance to achieve the general anesthetic state during surgery ("**maintenance** of anesthesia"). At the conclusion of surgery, the anesthetic gases are turned off, intravenous anesthetic agents are no longer administered, occasionally reversal medications are given when indicated, the patient is allowed to regain control of breathing until deemed safe to separate from the support of mechanical ventilation ("**emergence**"), the trachea is "extubated" and the patient taken to the Post Anesthesia Care Unit (PACU) for recovery. Finally, there is the post-operative visit in order to follow up for outcome, satisfaction and guidance for the future.

There are subspecialty-specific variations for pediatric, obstetric, cardiac and regional (nerve block) anesthesia, but the general theme is the same – it is a time-based experience of uncertainty for the patient and controlled, ideal operating conditions for the surgeon for an optimal result. One of the exquisite ironies is that time is imperceptible to the patient – and often too slow for the surgeon!

Standing guard over the beginning and end of this time for the patient is the anesthesiologist, warden of physiological homeostasis, defender of life-sustaining oxygenation of the vital organs, and keeper of the pharmacology arsenal of anesthetics. Peering at the past must include medical and surgical experiences as well as prior and current state of health. Living in the present, the anesthetist requires constant vigilance and mindfulness. Gazing into the future is the essential part of staying a step ahead of the numerous uncertainties that coexist with the surgical experience and the response of humans to it. Like Janus, looking at the past and the future are inseparable – fused together, as it were – for an anesthesiologist during the surgical experience. While all the other events and individuals are engaged in the contemporaneous surgical dance to the music of time, the anesthetist is the seneschal of the beginning and end.

***

In Act I, Scene 2 of *Othello*, Iago invokes the name of Janus after he fails to murder Othello. If not for Iago's two-faced cunning, Othello and Desdemona would probably have remained married and Cassio would have remained in power. Iago's schemes initiate the fall of each of the main characters and as the guide of the plot, he propels the story through inception, climax and finale. Janus' two-faced image is a convenient metaphor for Iago's character. Othello's characters believe him to have the best of intentions, calling him "honest Iago." However, Janus' image, used to highlight Iago's deception, is not what the Classical personification represented. Unlike Iago, Janus got a bum rap from Shakespeare.

Janus was indeed a god of opposites, but a dialectical god – beginnings and endings, exits and entrances, portals, doors and gates. He was the keeper of the calendar, welcoming the New Year ("January"). His two faces actually looked to the past and to the future. As the god of beginnings and endings, *he presided over time. He was there at the very beginning* – surnamed *divom deus*, an archaic form of Latin meaning the "the god of gods" – *and would be there at the very end.*

All events in Ancient Rome, routine and grand, began with an invocation to Janus. Every meal began with a request for his blessing. In the household, Janus' crucial role was *to prevent evil from crossing the threshold*. According to some, he was the *custodian* (janitor, derived from *janua* [L] for door) of the universe but, to all Romans, he was the god of the beginnings and endings, presiding over every entrance and departure. Because every door and passageway looks in two directions, Janus was two-faced – *Janus bifrons* – the god who looked both ways.

As a result of looking back at the past and being able to see the future, *Janus was able to select interventions to ameliorate the seemingly inevitable*. When Romulus, the founder of Rome, kidnapped the Sabine women, Janus caused a volcanic hot spring to erupt. The Sabines were buried alive in the resulting deadly hot water and ash mixture. Later on, however, the Sabines and Romans agreed to create a civilization together.

There was no comparable Greek deity with two faces. There was no other Roman deity that had a double aspect of this nature either. Janus was unique among all of the gods in western civilization in this respect, although Meslamta-ea, in the Babylonian epic Gilgamesh, was one of a pair of twin deities specifically associated with guarding doorways, *particularly the gateway to the underworld*, where they stood with bronze axes waiting to dismember the dead. In Egyptian mythology, the ferryman who carried souls into the land of the dead was, like Janus, also a two-faced deity known as Her-ef-ha-ef ("he whose face is behind him"). Usmu, the Babyloan messenger god, was also two-faced.

INTRODUCTION

Janus was involved in spatial transitions as well as transitions of time. He presided over doors, gates and boundaries. Several edifices between communities, especially Etrurians and Latins or Umbrians, are named after Janus. The most notable is the *Ianiculum*, which marked the access road to Etruria from Rome.

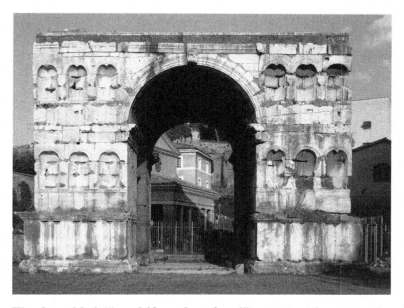

The four-sided ("quadrifons=four faced") structure known as the Arch of Janus (1st century CE). (Daderot, public domain, via Wikimedia Commons.)

***

Standing guard over the beginning and end of time.
Presiding over time.
Transitioning through space.
Being there at the very beginning and at the very end.
Preventing evil from crossing the threshold.
Selecting interventions to ameliorate the seemingly inevitable.
Guarding the gateway to the underworld.

The anesthetist watches over the patient, paying attention to time, space, and the transgressions of flesh and physiology that are the surgical experience. Starkly contrasting with Shakespeare's use of Janus as an icon of deception, the Classical image of Janus represents the passage of time, and with that passage in the context of patient care, the accumulation of knowledge, skill and wisdom acquired over that time. By being there during the surgical experience, from the beginning until the end, the anesthetist can make interventions that alter what could otherwise be mortally inevitable.

Within that very broad context, numerous values and traits integral to professionalism are cultivated and mobilized – which can be richly understood within the allegories of personification outlined so long ago.

Part I

THE HUMAN CONDITION

Everything was perfection ... until it was perfection no longer. This morality parable has existed since Original Sin in the Bible, and certainly in oral history before that. Everything was Paradise until the apple. In Hellenic mythology, everything was all right until Pandora's curiosity caused her to open the lid of the jar, letting disease and suffering out and only leaving Hope within. This set the stage for medicine, professionalism and the challenge of understanding diseases as well as the suffering, pain – and hope – that is the human condition.

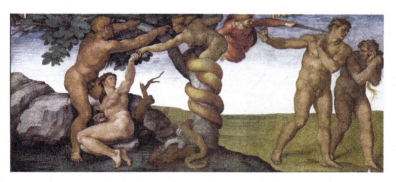

The Fall and Expulsion from the Garden of Eden. 1509–1510 Michaelangelo (1475–1564). (Michelangelo, public domain, via Wikimedia Commons.)

This fresco in the Sistine Chapel shows Adam and Eve to the left, the pair expelled from Paradise to the right, and the anthropomorphized Tree of Knowledge with the female

DOI: 10.1201/9781003201328-2

temptress in the center. To the left, the Garden of Eden is lush, to the right, barren. The story flows from left to right – Eve grasps the apple confidently, Adam intensely and selfishly. He senses his impending abandonment by God (Sistine Chapel, Vatican).

1
DISEASE: THE *NOSOI*

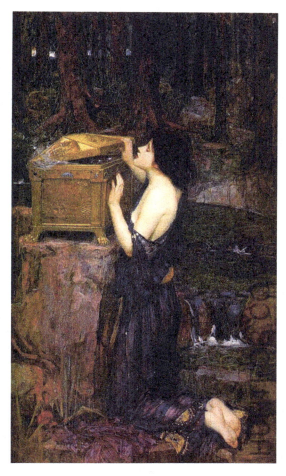

Pandora. 1896. Oil on canvas by John William Waterhouse (1849–1917). (John William Waterhouse, public domain, via Wikimedia Commons.)

DOI: 10.1201/9781003201328-3

For ere this (*the opening of Pandora's jar*) the tribes of men lived on earth remote and free from ills (*kakoi*) and hard toil (*ponoi*) and heavy sickness (*nosoi*) which bring the *Keres* (*Fates*) upon men; for in misery men grow old quickly. But the woman took off the great lid of the jar (*pithos*) with her hands and scattered all these and her thought caused sorrow and mischief to men.[1]

The use of fire, stone tools and speech paved the way for the development of family, extended family, tribe and, eventually, civilization. Although our forebears were consistently exposed to trauma, injuries, arthritis, and short lifespans, they probably were not exposed to widespread infectious diseases because they lacked the high population density required, a situation with which we are now all too familiar. In addition, because of the need to search for food, small groups did not remain in the same place for long enough to pollute water sources or accumulate the filth that attracts disease-producing insects. Moreover, hunter-foragers did not tend cattle and other tamed animals. Nomadic lifestyles continued until the end of the last Ice Age, around 12,000–10,000 years ago, when agriculture, the cultivation of plants and eventually animals in a fixed location gave rise to sedentary human civilization. Farming, planting, irrigation, and the rise of villages and towns followed – and with them, disease.

***

Zeus assigned Prometheus, the Titan of forethought, the task of creating the race of man, but Prometheus was despondent at man's lot, such as it was at the whim of the Gods. He therefore stole fire from the Gods to help man. Zeus, furious at this betrayal, commanded *Hephaistos* (L. *Vulcan*), the Greek god of artisans and craftsmen, to create the first woman.

As Hesiod relates:

> *Prometheus* outwitted him (*Zeus*) and stole the far-seen gleam of unwearying fire in a hollow fennel stalk. And Zeus who thunders on high was stung in spirit ... and he made an evil thing for men as the price of fire; for the very famous

(*Hephaistos*) formed of earth the likeness of a shy maiden as the son of *Kronos* willed. And the goddess bright-eyed *Athene* girded and clothed her with silvery raiment, and down from her head she spread with her hands an embroidered veil.[2]

The creation of *Pandora* ("All gifts") was a collaborative effort, as Hesiod further describes in *Works and Days*:

> (and other gods were instructed to bestow their gifts upon her.) And all obeyed Lord *Zeus*, the son of *Kronos*. The renowned strong smith modelled her figure of earth, in the likeness of a decorous young girl, as the son of *Kronos* had wished ... and (*Hermes*) put a voice inside her, and gave her the name of woman, *Pandora*, because all the gods who have their homes on Olympos had given her each a gift, *to be a sorrow to men* who eat bread.[3]

While Hephaistos mixed earth and water in order to fashion a "sweet, lovely maiden-shape" Athena taught her needlework and weaving, Aphrodite gave her grace, and Hermes gave her a "shameless mind and a deceitful nature."[4] Thus, it was inevitable that she, ironically known as "All-Gifts," would ultimately bestow misery and disease on man. Endowed with beauty and cunning, Pandora was herself gifted to *Prometheus'* younger brother *Epimetheus* as a bride. For his part, Zeus gave Pandora a storage jar (*pithos*) as a wedding gift, knowing that her nature would result in its opening, releasing the evil spirits contained within, which would plague mankind forever. Prometheus had warned his brother not to accept any gifts from Zeus but Epimetheus did not listen; he accepted Pandora, who promptly scattered the contents of her jar.

Catastrophic consequences to the opening of the jar followed:

> Pandora brings with her (a jar or box) containing burdensome toil and sickness that brings death to men, diseases and a myriad other pains.[4]

Hesiod further elaborates in *Works and Days*:

> Only Hope was left within her unbreakable house, she (Hope) *remained under the lip of the jar, and did not fly away.*

Before (she could), Pandora replaced the lid of the jar. This was the will of aegis-bearing Zeus the Cloudgatherer.[1]

What were the evils that flew out of Pandora's jar and how did they plague the health of mankind? Only a general reference to *Nosoi* – "diseases" – is provided in Greek mythology, despite the etymology of "nosology," that branch of medicine that deals with the classification of diseases. The specifics of these evils were better described in Roman mythology by their Latin names *Morbus, Lues, Pestis, Tabes and Macies*.

Morbus Gallicus (the "French Disease") is also known as syphilis, and was well recognized throughout ancient Europe. The use of the Latin "*Lues*" denoted disease, especially contagious disease. Syphilis was also known as Lues *venerea*, or simply, *Lues*. Clinically identifiable in primary, secondary and tertiary presentations, its initial presentation consisted of skin lesions and ultimately, if untreated, often progressed to neurological dysfunction including insanity. The *moral notion of punishment by disease* was reflected in the naming of syphilis itself by the Italian physician-poet Girolamo Fracastoro (1478?–1553), who wrote "*Syphilis, sive Morbus Gallicus*" ("Syphilis, or the French Disease").[5] It was an epic poem about a boy named Syphilus who insulted Apollo, and was in turn punished with the disease. He also added, at the end of the poem, two mythological tales written in the style of the Roman poet Ovid, giving supernatural accounts of the disease's origin and supposed cures, including mercury and guaiacum (a tree extract, the efficacy of which was disputed by his contemporary, Paracelsus 1493/4–1541). In so doing, Fracastoro offered Europeans a physical distraction and scapegoat by describing its introduction to Europe by the French. He also allowed the Church to distance itself from the disease (Rome had thousands of prostitutes at the time) concomitant with the Papal edict for sexual abstinence as treatment.[6] It is clear historically that syphilis itself was recognized long before. In 1025 the Persian physician Avicenna (980–1037) suggested the use of mercury for treating syphilis.

Similarly, Romans called epilepsy *morbus caducus* (the falling sickness) as well as *morbus comitialis* (disease of the assembly hall), *morbus sacer* (the sacred sickness) or *morbus demoniacus* (the demonic sickness). It was a Roman custom to shut down the public assembly (*comitia*) for ritual purification whenever any legislator experienced a seizure.[7,8]

Pestis is Latin for plague, or pestilence, an infectious disease caused by *Yersinia pestis*, a gram-negative rod-shaped bacterium. *Pestis*, as a personification of pestilence, plague, illness, sickness and disease, was also a Roman component of *Nosos/Nosoi*, and was portrayed either as a single individual *daemon* (ancient form of demon, or spirit), or as a number of *daimones*.[9]

Tabes denoted *wasting of the body* or a part of it. We are currently familiar with its description of a feature of tertiary syphilis, *tabes dorsalis*, a slowly progressive degeneration of the dorsal columns of the spinal cord and sensory nerve trunks resulting in impaired sensation and reflexes. The resulting movement disorder, known as locomotor ataxia, may appear 5 to 20 years after the initial syphilis infection. The typical gait of a tabetic patient is jerky and wide-based. *Tabes mesenterica* described tuberculosis of the mesenteric and retroperitoneal lymph nodes in children.

Finally, *macies* (L. *macer* – "meager or poor") denoted emaciation or atrophy.

In addition to the *Nosoi*, Virgil went on to describe the other evil spirits, many of which directly or indirectly affect disease as well as the all-too-human caregivers who treat disease:

Luctus (Grief) (L. Penthos)
Curae (Cares)
Morbi (Diseases) (L. Nosoi)
Senectus (Old Age) (L. Geras)
Metus (Fear) (L. Deimos)
Fames (Hunger) (L. Limos)
Egestas (Want) (L. Aporia)
Letum (Death) (L. Thanatos)
Labor (Toil) (L. Ponos)
Sopor (Sleep) (L. Hypnos)
Gaudia (the soul's guilty joys)
Bellum (War) (L. Polemos]
Eumenides [the Furies]
Discordia (Strife) (L. Eris)
Somnia (Dreams) (L. Oneiroi)

Why did all of these *daimones*, or spirits of misery, escape, and why was only Hope left behind? The role of Hope, *Elpis* (Ελπις), as the spiritual dialectic of Disease and Misery, was commented on by Aesop in Fables and offers a broader and more literary perspective:

> Zeus gathered all the useful things together in a jar and put a lid on it. He then left the jar in human hands. But man had no self-control and he wanted to know what was in that jar, so he pushed the lid aside, letting those things go back to the abode of the gods. So all the good things flew away, soaring high above the earth, and Hope was the only thing left. When the lid was put back on the jar, Hope was kept inside. That is why *Hope alone is still found among the people, promising that she will bestow on each of us the good things that have gone away.*[10]

This narrative is also less misogynistic than the traditional version by Hesiod two centuries earlier, in that Pandora does not open the box but rather "man" – which might have been Epimetheus, her husband, or the more generic "mankind."

In the justification of Zeus' punishment of man in the context of Pandora's jar, Aesop goes on to comment and clarify the balance of power between the Evils released and the Good that remained:

> The Good Things were too weak to defend themselves from the Bad Things, so the Bad Things drove them off to heaven. The Good Things then asked Zeus how they could reach mankind. Zeus told them that they should not go together all at once, only one at a time. This is why people are constantly besieged by Bad Things, since they are nearby, while Good Things come more rarely, since they must descend to us from heaven one by one.[10]

This moral message serves to show the reader that good things do not happen very often, while bad things happen to us all the time. The theme of punishment, original sin, guilt, and the "what have I done wrong" feeling as well as "what must I now do to make this evil / suffering / pain / bad luck go away" feeling occupies a large portion of the health care interaction and an even larger part of the sufferer's time away from the health care system.

The significance of Hope is further elaborated on by Aeschylus in Prometheus Bound:

> *Prometheus*: Yes, I caused mortals to *cease foreseeing their doom* (*Moros*).
> *Chorus*: Of what sort was the cure that you found for this affliction?
> *Prometheus*: I caused blind hopes (*Elpides*) to dwell within their breasts.
> *Chorus*: A great benefit was this you gave to mortals.[9]

***

To know the misery of Disease is also to recognize the strength of Hope, an underrepresented topic in medical education, and one that perhaps should be studied more seriously, along with disease. Maybe "Hope and Disease" should supplement "Health and Disease" as the dialectic Nosology and – Elpisiology? This concept has been suggested by Jerome Groopman in "The Anatomy of Hope.[11] While hope enters the conversation more frequently when anesthesiologists practice pain management and critical care, it is certainly part of the thoughts of every patient who is at the threshold of the anesthetic state, hoping for a cure, a restoration of function, and awakening.

References

1. Hesiod. *Works and Days*. www.theoi.com/Text/HesiodWorks Days. html. Accessed: 9/27/2016.
2. Hesiod. *The Homeric Hymns and Homerica. Theogony*. London, William Heinemann Ltd. Translated by: Evelyn-White H, 1914.
3. Hesiod. *Works and Days*. www.theoi.com/Text/HesiodWorks Days. html. Accessed: 9/27/16, 60 ff.
4. Hesiod. *Works and Days*. www.theoi.com/Text/HesiodWorks Days. html. Accessed: 9/27/16, 54 ff.
5. Fracastoro G. *Syphilis sive morbus gallicus*, 1530.
6. Di Cicco C. *History of Syphilis: A Night with Venus, a Lifetime with Mercury*, Amazon Digital Services LLC, 2011, p. 65.

7. Berger A. *Encyclopedic Dictionary of Roman Law.* Transactions of the American Philosophical Society (New Ser) 1953; 43: 333–809.
8. Aronson S. He hath the falling sickness. *Med Health RI* 1999; 82: 151–2.
9. Aeschylus. *Aeschylus I, Loeb Classical Library.* Edited by Capps E PT, Rouse WHD. London, W. Heinemann, 1922.
10. Aesop. *Aesop's Fables.* A new translation by Laura Gibbs, World's Classics, Oxford, Oxford University Press, 2008.
11. Groopman J. *The Anatomy of Hope.* New York, Random House. 2004.

2
HEALTH AND HEALING: THE *ASKLEPIADES*

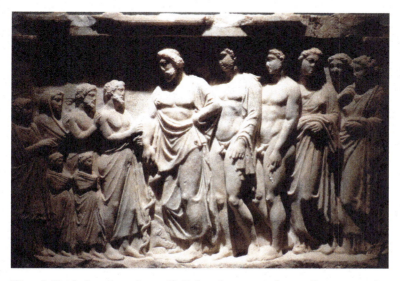

The *Asklepiades*. A votive relief showing mortal supplicants on the left, asking for help from *Asklepios* and his children. Close inspection reveals *Hygeia* standing behind *Asklepios*, almost in the shadows and barely visible; *Makhaon* and *Podalirios* stand to his right, then three goddesses, probably *Akeso*, *Iaso* and *Panakeia*.

"I swear by Apollo the physician, and Asklepios, and Hygieia and Panakea and all the gods and goddesses as my witnesses, that, according to my ability and judgment, I will keep this Oath and this contract…"[1]

This commencement oath to *Apollo* and his offspring marks the start of a doctor's professional life and is the traditional Western basis of a physician's professionalism. The promise of allegiance to Apollo and his family allowed the Ancients, via

DOI: 10.1201/9781003201328-4

personification, to afford us a trenchant view of early medical attitudes.[2,3]

***

Apollon

Apollon (L.: Apollo) was the god of truth as well as the god of light. In addition, as the god of the bow he could punish by inflicting illness with his arrows as well as heal and purify, hence his designation as physician. *Apollon* fell in love with the mortal *Koronis* (L.: Coronis), a princess of Thessaly.[*] While pregnant by *Apollon*, she was unfaithful with a mortal, *Iskhys*. *Apollon* complained to his sister *Artemis*, the goddess of the Hunt, who avenged her brother's insult by killing *Koronis* with her unerring arrows. *Apollon's* remorse led him to save the unborn child at *Koronis'* death, whom *Apollon* named *Asklepios* ("cut open").

Asklepios

The infant *Asklepios* (L.: Asclepius) was delivered as an apprentice, to *Kheiron* (L.: Chiron) the Centaur, wise as well as skilled in the use of herbs, incantations and cooling potions and from whom he learned medicine. *Asklepios* became skilled in surgery and the use of drugs, and has been regarded ever since as the founder of medicine:

> I begin to sing of Asclepius,
> son of Apollo and healer of sicknesses.
> In the Dotian plain[†] fair Coronis,
> daughter of King Phlegyas,
> bare him, a great joy to men, a soother of cruel pangs.[4]

The soothing of such cruel pangs was made possible because Athena gave *Asklepios* a magic potion made from the blood of the Gorgon.[‡] According to Apollodorus:

---

[*] An area in northern Greece bordering the Aegean Sea.
[†] Probably located in Thessaly. The reference "Dotian" is probably an honorific assigned to Phylegas' mother, Dotis.
[‡] A female creature in Greek mythology, from gorgós, which means dreadful. While descriptions of Gorgons vary, the term usually refers to any of the three sisters who had hair of living, venomous snakes, and a frightening gaze that turned those who beheld it to stone.

And having become a surgeon, and carried the art to a great pitch, he not only prevented some from dying, *but even raised up the dead*; for he had received from Athena the blood that flowed from the veins of the Gorgon, and while he used the blood that flowed from the veins on the left side for the bane of mankind, he used the blood that flowed from the right side for salvation, and by that means he raised the dead.[5]

Raising the dead, a great offense to *Hades*, the god of the Underworld, was aggravated by an *accusation of greed*. According to Pindar:

"But, alas!" he said, "even the lore of leech-craft[§] is enthralled by the love of gain; even he (*Asklepios*) was seduced by a splendid fee of gold displayed upon his palm, to bring back from death (*Hades*) one who was already its lawful prey. Therefore the son of Kronos (*Zeus*) with his hands hurled his shaft through both of them and quickly reft the breath from out their breasts for they were stricken with sudden doom by the gleaming thunderbolt."[6]

Followers of *Asklepios* were known as *Askelpiades*; the original *Asklepiades* were the family of *Asklepios*. His wife, *Epione* (Ἠπιόνη) (L.: Epione) was the goddess of the soothing of pain, which was the translation of her name. Together they had at least five daughters and three sons, all of whom personified various professional ideals.

The Daughters of Asklepios

Hygeia (L.: Hygea) was the goddess of *health, cleanliness, sanitation and disease prevention*. While her father was more directly associated with healing, *Hygeia* was associated with *the prevention of sickness and the continuation of good health*. The reference to *Hygeia* in the Orphic Hymns suggests the importance of health maintenance in the hierarchy of the children of *Asklepios*:[7]

and men without thy all-sustaining ease, find nothing useful, nothing form'd to please;

---
§ The art of healing.

Without thy aid, not Plutus' (Aides') self can thrive, nor man to much afflicted age arrive;
For thou alone of countenance serene, dost govern all things, universal queen.
Assist thy mystics with propitious mind, and far avert disease of ev'ry kind.

Her name is the source of the word hygiene. There are many representations of *Asklepios* and *Hygeia* together, the daughter often standing next to the seated father. In fact, they were so often portrayed together that some Ancient writers referred to *Hygeia* as the sister or wife of *Asklepios*.[8,9] She was typically depicted as a young woman feeding a large snake that was either wrapped around her body or drinking from a jar that she carried.

Iaso (L.: Iaso) was the goddess of *(complete) recuperation from illness*; her name is derived from the verb *iasthai*, "to heal." She is depicted as gazing into a mirror, *as if to confirm that recuperation was equivalent to status quo ante*.

Akeso (L.: Aceso) was the goddess of healing (wounds) and curing (illness). Unlike her sisters, she represented the *process of curing rather than the cure itself*; hence she was the goddess of recovery.

Aglaia (L.: Aglaea) was the *goddess of natural beauty*. Her genealogy is confusing, because according to a variety of sources, she was part of multiple lineages. Hesiod described her as the youngest of the three Graces[10] while Pausanias mentioned *Koronis* as a maternal possibility.[11]

Panakeia (L.: Panacea) was the goddess of healing and cures. She was said to have a poultice or potion with which she healed the sick. This brought about the concept of the *panacea* in medicine.

Meditrina (L.: Meditrina) was the keeper of the serpent of Asklepios and is portrayed in a limestone bas relief. The setting is unclear, but it may be a pharmacy, based on the presence of some specific tools and her *recognition as the goddess of medicine (medications)*.

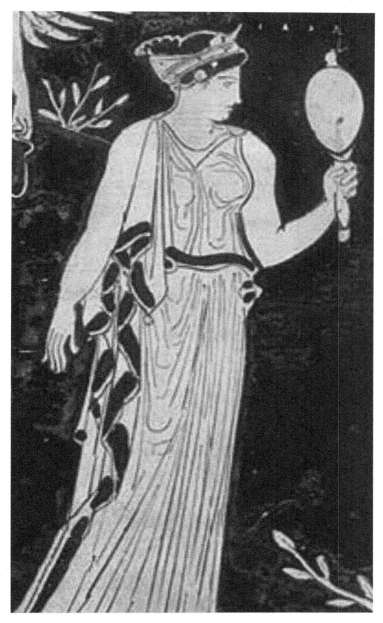

Iaso. Goddess of recuperation from illness. Cropped image of Iaso staring at herself in a mirror. From a Greek urn; c. 400 BCE. (The Cadmus Painter, public domain, via Wikimedia Commons.)

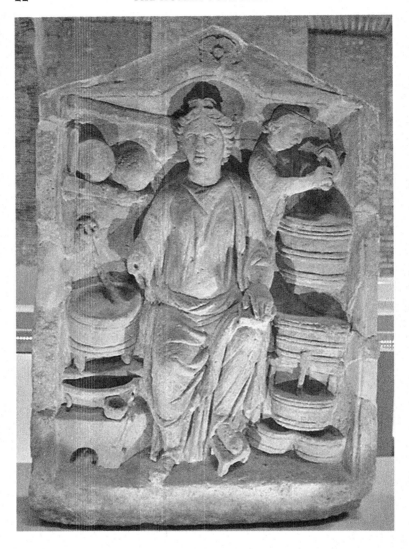

Meditrina. Goddess of medicine, perhaps pharmacy. Seated in the center, among casks and bottles, *Medetrina* is flanked by a smaller figure with a mortar and pestle and another stirring a mixture in a vat over a low heater. Roman Gaul. Found in Grand (Vosges), 2nd century CE. Le Muse Departemental d'art Ancien et Contemporain; Epinal (France). (Carole Raddato from Frankfurt, Germany, CC BY-SA 2.0, via Wikimedia Commons.)

The Sons of *Asklepios*

Makhaon (L.: Machaon), king of Tricca,** was a *master surgeon*, recognized as such in the Iliad, which also reported his wounding and incapacitation by Paris. Both he and his brother *Podaleirios* (L.: Podalirius) the second of the kings of Tricca, known as a diagnostician *(a healer of "internal" diseases)*, took part in the Trojan War. Arctinus the poet expressed the differences in their specialties:

> For their father himself, the glorious Earthshaker, gave them both honors, but one he made more renowned than the other. To the one he gave *more agile hands* to draw the darts from the flesh and to heal all wounds; to the other he gave the power *to know accurately in his heart all matters that are unseen*, and to heal things incapable of healing. He first understood the eyes flashing forth like lightning and the depressed mind of the mad Ajax.[12]

Telesphoros (L.: Telesphorus), the last of the sons of Asklepios and Epione, is depicted as a boy serving together with his sister Hygeia. He is typically shown as a small, almost childlike figure, in a hooded cloak and is generally thought of as symbolizing *recovery from illness* as his name means "the accomplisher," "bringer of completion" or "convalescence." However, alternate interpretations have been offered, included "finisher," which could mean the *Classical alternative to convalescence – death*. That he is not portrayed in the earlier bas relief of the *Asklepiades* is in keeping with the timing of his addition to the Asklepian legend, for which there is no physical evidence until about 200 CE.

***

Professionals are more than just experts. This distinction was suggested by the Ancients in the identification of *Apollon* as the first physician, although not necessarily the father of medicine. The difference is subtle but important – while *Apollon* had curative as well as intentionally harmful or lethal powers, *Asklepios* lacked the threatening capability of *Apollon* and moreover incorporated

---

** An ancient city in Thessaly.

additional aspects of the learned professions.†† This set the stage for values that we now acknowledge as professional obligations – expertise, lifelong learning, compassion, trust, responsibility and obligation to the greater society.

Having relatively little in the way of medications, physicians relied primarily on herbals in the hope of rejuvenating or restoring health before moving along to their next destination. *Apollon* the father, *Asklepios* the son and *Hygeia* the daughter are often portrayed with a single serpent next to them. The significance of the snake and staff, known as the *asklepian*, has been subject to various interpretations. The staff was thought to reflect the physician's itinerary. The shedding of the snakeskin and its renewal is emphasized as symbolizing rejuvenation and regeneration. Although there is some controversy about the use of the term,[13] one view of anesthesiology practice is as an ongoing resuscitation. In several countries, anesthesiology departments incorporate "reanimation" into their title.

Other assessments interpret the serpent as the expression of the dialectic of the physician, who deals with life and death, sickness and health. Indeed, drugs that can help as well as harm are the daily province of the anesthesiologist. The Ancients also recognized this linguistically; the term *pharmakon* meant "drug," "medicine" and "poison" in ancient Greek, hence the significance especially of *Meditrina* in the *Asklepiades*. Products derived from the bodies of snakes were known to have medicinal properties in ancient times, which could, if overdosed, be poisonous. In Greece, plants were used not only for healing, but also as a means of inducing death either through suicide or execution.[14]

No anesthetic is without risk, and all anesthetized patients must recover. To the *Asklepiades*, "recovery" was not only a *process* but also a *destination* as well as an expectation of *restoration to a pre-illness state*. Three of the *Asklepiades* were dedicated to these nuanced concepts of recovery. The language used to describe the roles of *Asklepios* and his family had many subtle

---

†† Traditionally, the practice of law, medicine and theology, requiring advanced knowledge after a prolonged course of specialized instruction and study. The first requirement is that the knowledge be of an advanced type. Second, it must be knowledge in a field of science or learning, distinguishing the professions from the mechanical arts. There is also a requirement for literacy.

and contextually rich meanings. Many of our interactions with patients are layered in this fashion, superimposed on the uncertainties[3] that they acknowledge during the informed consent process. When patients ask "when will I be awake," the definitions may be different depending upon whether we are answering according to process ("you will be talking to us in the post-anesthesia care unit (PACU) and we can give you juice and crackers") or a baseline, non-medicated state ("don't make any business decisions until tomorrow"). The notion that a perfectly safe and effective anesthetic or combination of anesthetic medications would provide a "panacea," a universal elixir or magic bullet, is not credible – therefore adding to the uncertainty of the anesthetized state.

There is often a price to be paid for medical and surgical intervention – there is rarely a free lunch. The marriage of *Asklepios* and *Epione*, metaphorically pairing "cutting open" with "the soothing of pain," recognized the pairing of surgery and pain relief since Ancient times. Ironically though, it is Hygeia, not *Epione*, whom we see most often paired with *Asklepios*, standing by his side or behind him, giving equal weight to the curative / palliative as well as the preventive role of health care. Politically and economically expedient as well, this hierarchy may have intentionally emphasized the importance of attracting not only the sick to the cult of *Asklepios*, but also the healthy. To complement this interpretation, the juxtaposition of *Telesphoros* as a diminutive, cloaked figure in (unequal) balance to *Asklepios* and *Hygeia* suggests that *Telesphoros* may indeed have represented the blessing of death, the Classical view of another acceptable outcome of healing, while not overemphasizing death as an equivalent choice. *Hygeia* and *Telesphoros*, therefore, may have represented "both sides" of *Asklepios*.[15]

Despite the progress made toward egalitarianism between the medical establishment and patients, there remains a significant gulf between the world of the suppliant and that of the expert. The manner of depiction in the *Asklepiades* bas relief is worthy of mention. First of all, *Machaon* and *Podalirius* are shown nude while *Asklepios* is dressed. Nudity was the traditional presentation for Greek hero-gods, a figurative reflection of perfection and a literal reflection of "nothing to hide." We currently and colloquially call this "transparency" in the patient–doctor relationship.

The clothed *Asklepios*, certainly more traditional in current times, is historically more in keeping with the wandering nature of the Ancient physician, encountering a wide range of families in many different locations – it was important to dress properly. That the gods were viewed as greater than the suppliants is underscored by the differences in their size, bearing, gaze and the mortals' support for each other through touch, contrasted with the gods' individual stances. As gods, they scarcely needed mutual support.

***

What purpose was served by the portrayal of the *Asklepiades* as a family and the children of *Asklepios* as children, rather than as values attached to *Asklepios* himself? One interpretation is that by separating the qualities of healing practice from the act of healing itself, more room was left for the "miraculous" cures of *Asklepios*. While it is easy to think that health and cure should be related, and in fact this is what we are trying to integrate into current medical practice with the concept of "wellness," separating the concepts allows a basic dilemma to be avoided – why should the sustainer of health also need to provide cures? This duality remains a conceptual challenge in anesthesiology practice. Anesthetists are well familiar with the "zero-error" and "complete reversibility" expectation that all patients will be returned to their *status quo ante* after the anesthetic is completed, and the difficulty in adjudicating less than completely *status quo ante* outcomes remains a challenge in perioperative care. The creation of a "family" allowed the physician the separation required to examine values beyond those assigned to the healing role, and in this manner, enabled independent consideration of the soothing of pain, hygiene, recovery, convalescence, cure, medicines and preservation of the hope for an all-encompassing medicine. In numerous anesthetic pharmacology papers and textbooks, this is typically called "the ideal anesthetic," a euphemism for a panacea.

A word about *Hygeia* – a proxy for wellness – for the professional. In accordance with the ethical guidelines set forth by the American Society of Anesthesiologists, anesthesiologists must maintain their "physical and mental health and special sensory capabilities."[16] Similar recognition is made by every medical specialty board. Unfortunately, the emphasis on impairment labeling, intervention and post-intervention monitoring of state medical Boards' Physician Health committees provides little guidance and support for developing and sustaining a healthier lifestyle, nor an infrastructure for research and education. In 1979, then Surgeon General Dr. Julius Richmond, a pediatrician–psychiatrist, provided the first national wellness agenda: "Healthy People – Surgeon General's Report on Health Promotion and Disease Prevention." A new ten-year plan is published decennially; "Healthy People 2030" was just published recognizing 355 public health objectives that have ten-year targets and are associated with evidence-based interventions.

Apollon, Asklepios and the original *Asklepiades* set the tone for the Hippocratic oath, one of the cornerstones of medical professionalism. The personifications of health (hygiene and prevention), medicine (pharmacy), universally applicable treatment (panacea), the process of healing (recovery) as well as the endpoint or completion of healing, and lastly, beauty and a return to a stable state remain cornerstones of anesthetic practice. After all, who does not see the allure of an anesthetic well done, leading to a "beautiful" result?

References

1. Hippocrates. *The Hippocratic Oath: National Library of Medicine*, National Institutes of Health. www.nlm.nih.gov/hmd/greek/greek_oath.html.
2. Bailey J. Asklepios: ancient hero of medical caring. *Ann Int Med*. 1996; 124(2): 257–63.
3. Holzman R. Uncertainty by choice: anesthesia and the children of night. *J Clin Anesth* 2002; 14: 46–51.
4. Anonymous. *The Homeric Hymns and Homerica*. Cambridge, MA, Harvard University Press, 1914. www.perseus.tufts.edu.
5. Apollodorus. *The Library of Greek Mythology*. Frazer SJG, editor. Lawrence, KS, Coronado Press, 1975.
6. Pindar. *The Complete Odes* New York, Oxford University Press, 474 BC [updated 2007. 186]. www.perseus.tufts.edu.
7. Athanassakis A. *The Orphic Hymns: Text, Translation and Notes*. Missoula, MT, Scholars Press, 1977, 146 p.
8. Jayne W. *The Healing Gods of Ancient Civilizations*. New Haven, Yale University Press, 1925.

9. Taylor T. *The Hymns of Orpheus, Translated from the Original Greek: With a Preliminary Dissertation on the Life and Theology of Orpheus*. London, T. Payne, 1792, 227 p.
10. Hesiod. *Theogony*. Cambridge, MA, Harvard University Press; 1914. http://omacl.org/Hesiod/hymns.html.
11. Pausanias. *Description of Greece*. Cambridge, MA, Harvard University Press, 1918, ix. 35, para. 1 p.
12. Sigerist H. *Archaic Medicine in Greece: Homeric Medicine. A History of Medicine: Early Greek, Hindu, and Persian Medicine*. Department of the History Medicine, Yale University, no. 38, 2. New York, Oxford University Press, 1961, p 32.
13. Van Norman G. Do-not-resuscitate orders during anesthesia and urgent procedures: University of Washington School of Medicine, 1998, http://depts.washington.edu/bioethx/topics/dnrau.html.
14. Holzman R. The Legacy of Atropos, the Fate Who Cut the Thread of Life. *Anesthesiology* 1998; 89(1): 241–9.
15. Weiss M. Telesphoros: neglected son of Asklepios. *J Paleopathol.* 1993; 5: 53–9.
16. Committee on Ethics ASoA. *Guidelines for the Ethical Practice of Anesthesiology*. Chicago, IL, American Society of Anesthesiologists, 2013.

3

UNCERTAINTY: *NYX* AND HER CHILDREN

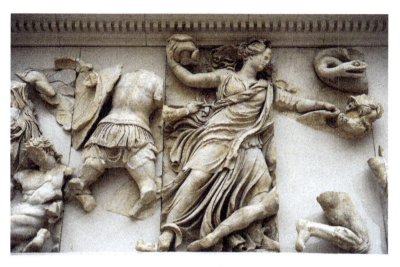

Nyx (Night), born of Khaos, was the primordial goddess of the night and the mother of *Hypnos* (sleep) *Thanatos* (death) and *Morpheus* (dreams) as well as the Fates *Klotho, Lachesis and Atropos*. Here, she holds a vessel surrounded with snakes that she uses as a weapon against a giant. (From the North frieze, Gigantomachy frieze, Pergamon Museum, Berlin.)

Embarking upon the surgical experience, anxious patients and their families face the risks of the anesthetic and procedure, the discomfort of recovery and the uncertainty of outcome. More than an imprecise understanding of the anesthetized state is at work here; historical evidence, pervasive in recorded art and literature, bears witness to the entwining of fear, loss of personal control and mortality with the perceived continuum of sleep, dreams, drug-induced stupor and death. It is at this juncture of sleep, dreams and "reanimation," as anesthesiology is known in some of the world, that these boundaries become blurred not by our imperfect understanding of the science but rather by the patient's and anesthesiologist's mutual feelings of uncertainty. The ancient Greeks personified these states as siblings, the children of the goddess Night (*Nyx*): Sleep (*Hypnos*), Dreams (*Morpheus*), Death (*Thanatos*), and the Fates, *Klotho, Lachesis* and *Atropos*.

***

Nyx (L.: Nox)

Born of *Khaos, Nyx* herself was mother to many of the "darker" gods and spirits – *Momus* (blame), *Moros* (fate), *Thanatos* (death), *Hypnos* (sleep), the *Onerois* (dreams), the *Hesperides* (the evening nymphs), *Nemesis* (retribution), *Apate* (deception) and *Eris* (strife). Homer referred to her as the "subduer of gods and men." She also gave birth to the stars, according to the Orphic hymns. In particular, *Nyx*'s power even over the gods was evident in the Iliad, following the sleep induced by *Hypnos* over *Zeus* at *Hera*'s bidding:

> (*spoken by Hypnos*) "That time I laid to sleep the brain in Zeus ... but Zeus awakened in anger and beat the gods up and down his house, looking beyond all others for me, and would have sunk me out of sight in the sea from the bright sky had not *Nyx* (Night) who has power over gods and men rescued me. I reached her in my flight, and Zeus let be, though he was angry, in awe of doing anything to swift Nyx' displeasure."[1]

Hypnos (Sleep) (L. *Somnus*)

Homer (ca. 9th–8th century BCE) referred to *Hypnos* as the "brother of Death":

Then, taking wing from Athos'* lofty steep,
She speeds to Lemnos,† o'er the rolling deep,
And seeks the cave of Death's half brother, Sleep.[2]

In works of art, the brothers *Hypnos* and *Thanatos* (Death) often slumbered together, holding inverted torches in their hands. Ironically, Sleep was acknowledged as the more powerful because of his ability to conquer even the gods who were immune to Death. In *Hera*'s‡ paean to *Hypnos*:

> Hypnos, mighty lord of all gods and of all men,
> If you ever listened to my words, and you now
> Would obey, I shall ever be grateful to you.
> Lull to sleep the bright eyes under the brows of Zeus,
> For me, as soon as I lay by his side in love.

She acknowledged this special status of Hypnos, who nevertheless, demurred:

> Hera, Queenly goddess
> Any other of the immortal gods, I might
> Easily lull to sleep,
> But I will not go near to Zeus, son of Cronus,§
> Nor lull him to sleep, unless he bids me himself
> For I was taught well on another occasion
> When I charmed the mind of Zeus, the aegis** bearer,
> With sound sleep
> But when awakened he was wrath,
> Flung the gods about, in the hall, searching for me

---

* Mount Athos, a mountain in Chalcidice, Macedonia.
† Greek island in the northeast Aegean Sea, considered to have been only inhabited by women.
‡ The queen of the Olympian gods, eldest daughter of Kronos and Rhea and wife and sister of Zeus.
§ Kronos, the son of Uranus and Gaia and the youngest of the 12 Titans. His wife was Rhea and their offspring were Demeter, Hestia, Hera, Hades, Poseidon and Zeus.
** The shield of Zeus, later associated with Athena.

Above all, and would have hurled me into the deep,
To be seen no more, had not mother Night saved me.[3]

This passage suggests that *both the commencement of and emergence from sleep could have dire consequences* – a warning for anesthesiologists and their patients. In a similar fashion, sacrifices to Hypnos were made in the sanctuary of the Muses at Corinth, while professing:

> Hypnos is the god that is dearest to the Muses.[4]

Thanatos (Death)

Drawing a stark contrast between the brothers, Hesiod's (8th century BCE) poetry called Death "pitiless" and Sleep "kind:"

> ... the children of dark Night have their dwellings
> Sleep and Death, awful gods
> ... the former of them roams peacefully over the earth
> and the sea's broad back and is kindly to men;
> But the other has a heart of iron
> and his spirit within him is pitiless as bronze:
> Whomever of men he has once seized he holds fast:
> and he is hateful even to the deathless gods.[5]

Yet the feared Thanatos was also seen as a healer, the *iatros*[††] *kakon*[‡‡] *who, rather than seizing men against their will, released them from the burden of mortal life.* Euripdes' (ca. 480–406 BCE) Hippolytos, in his last painful moments, prayed that Death would come to him as a healer:

> Oh! Oh! And now the pain, the pain, comes over me.
> Let me go, wretched man that I am, and may Death come to me as healer.
> Kill me, kill the wretch that I am!
> I long for a two-edged blade to cut my life in two and lay it to rest.[6]

[††] One who heals, physician or surgeon.
[‡‡] Worthless, sorry, unskilled.

Morpheus (Dreams)

Morpheus, also recognized as the son as well as the prime minister of Hypnos, was the god of dreams. He was worshipped together with *Hypnos* and *Thanatos* in the sanctuary of *Asklepios* in Corinth, where:

> There were statues of Oneiros[§§] and Hypnos, surnamed Bountiful, lulling to sleep a lion.[7]

A crown of poppies graced his head and in his hand he held a goblet full of poppy juice, which he gently shook to induce a state of drowsiness – according to him, the perfection of bliss. It fell to *Morpheus*, as the prime minister of *Hypnos*, to guard his charge and watch over his slumbers, preventing anyone from troubling his sleep. The pharmacist Friedrich Sertürner derived the name of the opiate drug morphine from the name *Morpheus*.

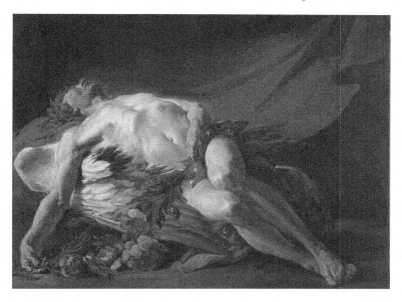

[§§] Morpheus was one of four sons of Hypnos, collectively known as the Oneroi – *Icelus* (dreams of humans), *Morpheus* (shaping dreams), *Phobetor* (frightening dreams of beasts), and *Phantasos* (apparitions).

Morpheus. c. 1771 Jean-Bernard Restout (1732–1797) (Jean-Bernard Restout, public domain, via Wikimedia Commons.)

The inspiration for this painting may have been Ovid's *Metamorphoses*, which described the god of sleep as living in a cave with sleep-inducing poppies at the entrance.

The Fates – *Klotho, Lachesis* and *Atropos*

The daughters of *Nyx* sat near *Hades'* throne. *Klotho*, the youngest, spun the thread of life, throughout which bright and dark lines were woven. *Lachesis*, the second, twisted the thread; under her fingers it was alternately strong, then weak. *Atropos*, the third sister, cut the thread of life with oversized shears – an intimation that before long, another soul would find its way into the kingdom of *Hades*. These personifications of the uncertainties of life were eloquently described in the Spindle Song by Sir Walter Scott (1771–1832):

> Twist ye, twine ye! even so,
> Mingle shades of joy and woe,
> Hope, and fear, and peace, and strife,
> In the thread of human life.[8]

It was Hesiod who suggested that the Fates were the daughters of Night:

> And Night bore hateful Doom and black Fate and Death.
> and she bore Sleep and the tribe of Dreams ...
> Also she bore the Destinies and ruthless avenging Fates,
> Klotho and Lachesis and Atropos, who give men at their
>   birth both evil and good to have.[9]

as did Aeschuylus (525–456 BCE):

> you, divine Fates, our sisters by one mother,
>   divinities who distribute justly, who have a share in
>   every home,
>   and whose righteous visitations press heavily at every season[10]

Even among the immortal Olympian gods, the Fates were feared because they represented uncertainty:

> They also knew, but seldom revealed, what would be the fate of each Olympian god. Even Zeus feared them for that reason.[11]

***

For the Ancients, sleep and dreams connected the physical to the metaphysical world. Revelations were thought to pass to mortals through the mechanism of dreams. During his dream, the patient sleeping in the Amphiareion[†††] received advice or curative instructions about his problem, similar to the revelations of those sleeping within the Asklepieion or the sanctuary of the Muses. These beliefs helped to explicate the inexplicable. Perhaps anesthesiologists, after a fashion, invoke the same model when using the less threatening "sleep" as a proxy for controlled unconsciousness, analgesia, and ventilatory and circulatory support. Unfortunately, the anesthetized state provides no guarantee of dreams, let alone their utility for planning one's future.

Anesthesiologists carefully counsel patients about the recovery from anesthesia. Ironically, the hope that sleep would only be a temporary state, distinct from its allegorical siblings, had been pleaded by Samuel Daniel (1562–1619), long before modern surgical anesthesia:

> Care-Charmer Sleep, son of the sable Night,
> Brother to Death, in silent darkness born,
> Relieve my languish, and restore the light;
> With dark forgetting of my care return.[12]

while John Donne (1572–1631) challenged Death with a caustic yet intriguing comparison to his siblings:

> Thou'rt slave to fate, chance, kings, and desperate men,
> And dost with poison, war, and sickness dwell;
> And poppy or charms can make us sleep as well
> And better than thy stroke. Why swell'st thou then?[13]

[†††] Sleeping chamber named after the legendary healer and king of Argos, who was worshipped as a god.

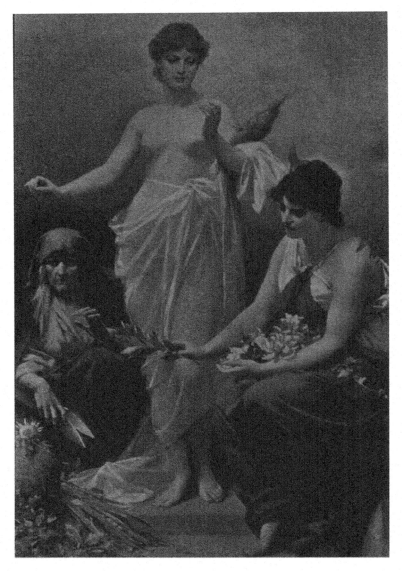

The Fates, Klotho, Lachesis and Atropos (After Paul Thumann, public domain, via Wikimedia Commons.)

William Shakespeare (1564–1616) intentionally blurred the Sleep/Death euphemism in Hamlet's soliloquy. He advocated the relief brought by the sleep of death, much as the Ancients had portrayed Death as a healer:

> To die: to sleep;
> No more; and, by a sleep to say we end
> The heart-ache and the thousand natural shocks
> That flesh is heir to, 'tis a consummation
> Devoutly to be wish'd.[14]

Nor is the uncertainty about the anesthetic state limited to articulate adults. The uncertainty and fear are intertwined at a young age when children are educated with the Child's Bedtime Prayer:

> Now I lay me down to sleep,
> I pray the Lord my soul to keep;
> If I should die before I wake,
> I pray the Lord my soul to take.[15]

Imagine then the fear lurking behind the uncertainty of the innocent preanesthetic question asked by a five-year-old – "so how do you know I'm asleep and not dead?" Children commonly ask the questions that adults fear to ask.

Unlike Sleep, Death was generally overlooked in Greek literature (as it often is in medical conversations). The deliberate omission of Death may have been motivated in part by the same superstitious caution that routinely prevented mention of his name as well as by viewing death as a continuum of life. Olympian politics may also have played a role; because Thanatos was the god of the dead while Hades was the Olympian king or ruler of the dead, the stature of Hades, brother of Zeus and Poseidon and son of Kronos, was more important than that of Thanatos. This may also fit in with the notion that Sleep is actually the more powerful of the two (*vide supra*) because of the elements of uncertainty yet control, a dialectic not dissimilar to the one that anesthesiologists face daily. Despite the uncertainty of both the patient and the practitioner, that uncertainty can be controlled to a large extent by making optimal choices and monitoring in the operating room and critical care unit.

Don't take the rather benign word "sleep" for granted in medical conversations – we (meaning everyone) use "sleep" as a proxy for "controlled drug-induced unconsciousness" all the time. The consistently dyadic portrayal of the more forgiving Hypnos seemed to soften the impact of the accompanying Thanatos, a euphemism we preserve to this day. Sleep and Death were shown as children on the Chest of Kypselos (Elis), held, one in each arm, by their nurse, Night.[7] All three were labeled, but Pausanias' comments suggested that their identities would be obvious without the labels. One of the children was white, the other black. The white child was sleeping ("*katheudonta*") while the black one was "like one asleep" ("*katheudonti eoikota*"), suggesting that the former was "true Sleep" and the latter Death, who was "like Sleep." The construction of the language is redolent of the Greek word for "a not-feeling" pain – *anaisthesia*.[16–18]

***

Anesthesiologists sometimes have difficulty discussing uncertainties with patients. In non-anesthetic medical interventions, consequences and side effects of treatment, such as pain, infection, adverse reactions to an antibiotic or nausea with cancer chemotherapeutic drugs, are accepted with reluctant resignation. Ironically, accompanying the expectation of complete reversibility and recovery from anesthesia is the typical anesthesia consent form phrasing of (rare) "severe adverse drug reactions, brain damage or death." What makes this worthy of reflection is the popularly widespread and deeply visceral uncertainty about sleep, dreams and death, the daily terrain of the anesthesiologist.

There are suggestions that uncertainty may not be recognized by all anesthesiologists as a part of the process of anesthesia and these anesthesiologists appear to function with some inflexibility, according to a preconceived plan.[19] Jerome Kassirer has pithily pointed out that a physician's task "is not to attain certainty but rather to reduce the level of diagnostic uncertainty enough to make optimal therapeutic decisions."[20] The patient safety movement, having had its embryology in the acknowledgment of the uncertainties of anesthesiology and the multifactorial nature of anesthesia-related accidents and mishaps,[21] has pioneered an approach to patient-centered safety through simulation training, in itself a calculus of uncertainty.[22]

The Ancients cloaked in mystery events that occurred in the natural world, but even when evidence-based data provides robust probabilities for outcome, a person's soul is still not reassured when uncertainty is encountered. It may be through the acknowledgement of that ancient mythology by patient and practitioner that the way is paved to better come to grips with this most challenging and human aspect of our craft.

References

1. Homer. *Iliad*. Chicago, University of Chicago Press. Translated by: Lattimore R, 1961.
2. Homer. *The Iliad of Homer* 3rd ed. London, B. Lintot. Translated by: Pope A, 1732.
3. Homer. *The Iliad of Homer* 3rd ed. London, B. Lintot. Translated by: Pope A, 1732.
4. Pausanias. *Description of Greece*. Cambridge, MA, Harvard University Press. Translated by: Jones W, Omerod, H, 1931.
5. Hesiod. *Hesiod's Theogony*. Cambridge, MA, Focus Information Group. Translated by: Caldwell R, 1987.
6. Euripides. *Hippolytus*. Warminster, Aris & Phillips. Translated by: Halleran M, 1995.
7. Pausanias. *Description of Greece*. Cambridge, MA, Harvard University Press. Translated by: Jones W, Omerod, H, 1931.
8. Scott W. *Guy Mannering*. Edinburgh, Edinburgh University Press, 1999.
9. Hesiod. *Hesiod's Theogony*. Cambridge, MA, Focus Information Group. Translated by: Caldwell R, 1987.
10. Aeschylus. *The Eumenides*, xvi. Englewood Cliffs, NJ, Prentice-Hall. Translated by: Lloyd-Jones H, 1970.
11. Graves R. *Greek Gods and Heroes*. New York, Dell Publishing Co. Inc, 1960.
12. Daniel S. *Poems and a Defence of Rhyme*. Chicago, University of Chicago Press, 1965.
13. Donne J. Death. *The Oxford Book of English Verse, 1250–1900*. Edited by Quiller-Couch A. Oxford, Clarendon Press, 1921, pp 108.
14. Shakespeare W. *Hamlet, Prince of Denmark: The Complete Works of William Shakespeare*. Edited by Craig W. London, H. Milford, 1916, pp 1350 Act III. Scene I, 69–73.
15. Leonis E. *A Child's Bedtime Prayer, The New England Primer*, Twentieth century reprint edition. Boston, Ginn & Company, 1784.
16. Askitopoulou H, Ramoutsaki I, Konsolki E. Analgesia and anesthesia: etymology and literary history of related Greek words. *Anesth Analg* 2000; 91: 486–91.

17. Holzman R. The legacy of Atropos, the fate who cut the thread of life. *Anesthesiology* 1998; 89: 241–9.
18. Rey R. *The History of Pain*. Cambridge, Harvard University Press, 1995.
19. Klemola U, Norros L. Analysis of the clinical behaviour of anaesthetists: recognition of uncertainty as a basis for practice. *Medical Education* 1997; 31: 449–56.
20. Kassirer J. Our stubborn quest for diagnostic certainty, a cause of excessive testing. *N Engl J Med* 1989; 320: 1489–91.
21. Gaba D, Maxwell M, DeAnda A. Anesthetic mishaps: breaking the chain of accident evolution. *Anesthesiology* 1987; 66: 670–6.
22. Holzman R, Cooper J, Gaba D, Philip J, Small S, Feinstein D. Anesthesia crisis resource management: real-life simulation training in operating room crises. *Journal of Clinical Anesthesia* 1995; 7: 675–87.

4

SAFETY: *SOTERIA*

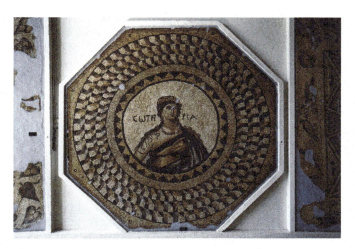

***Soteria*, portrayed as a woman wearing a laurel wreath crown, a symbol of victory, was the Greek goddess of safety, deliverance and preservation from harm.**

Anesthesiologists were founders of the modern patient safety movement. With the publication of "To Err is Human" in 2000,[1] the Institute of Medicine established a broad patient safety agenda for the twenty-first century. This followed *by almost 25 years* the landmark publication "Preventable Anesthesia Mishaps: A Study of Human Factors"[2] and the establishment in 1985 of the Anesthesia Patient Safety Foundation, the first patient safety-centered group in organized medicine. Yet *primum non nocere*, "first, do no harm," has been a cornerstone of medical non-maleficence for millennia.

Safety is far more than the absence or mitigation of risk. Advances in medical care are ultimately a balance between safety, caution and vigilance as well as strength, courage and daring.

THE HUMAN CONDITION

***

There is little written about *Soteria*, the Greek goddess of safety, deliverance and preservation from harm. Her male counterparts were the spirit *Soter* and the god *Dionysos Soter*. *Soteria* was portrayed as a woman wearing a laurel wreath crown, a symbol of victory. Soteriology is the academic study of salvation. In Roman mythology, *Soteria* was known as *Salus* (Preservation); however, *Salus*'s domain was characterized by physical wellbeing and health ("salutary") rather than safety, in the sense of security. The (Greek) Bible's use of *Soteria* reflects a more pious etymology, as the word is used to mean "fourfold salvation: saved from the penalty, power, presence and most importantly the pleasure of sin."[3] Salvation (Latin: *salvatio*) is *the act of being saved or protected from harm*[4] or *being saved or delivered from some dire situation*. This introduces a dialectic of safety and heroism.

According to Pausanias:

> In Aigion in Akhaia (Aegium in Achaea)[*] they also have a sanctuary of Soteria (Safety). Her image may be seen by none but the priests, and the following ritual is performed. They take cakes of the district from the goddess and throw them into the sea, saying that they send them to Arethousa[†] at Syrakousa (Syracuse).[5]

Pausanias referred to *Soteria* several times again:

> Eurypylos (the hero of the Trojan War) opened the chest containing a sacred idol of Dionysos, saw the image, and forthwith on seeing it went mad. He continued to be insane for the greater part of the time, with rare lucid intervals ...[6]
>
> There is a sanctuary (in Patrai in Akhaia [Patrae in Achaea]) with an image of stone. It is called the sanctuary of Soteria (*Deliverance*), and the story is that it was originally founded by Eurypylos on being cured of his madness.[7]

reminiscent of the subtle meanings of the Greek *Soteria* and the Latin *Salvatio*.

---

[*] Aigio, also known as Aegion is a town in Achaea, West Greece
[†] Arethousa was one of the Nereids and the nymph of the famous well Arethusa in the island of Ortygia near Syracuse. Virgil referred to her as the divinity who inspired pastoral poetry.

The laurel wreath crown worn by *Soteria* underscores the association of victory with safety and the deliverance from harm. Images of Apollo feature his wearing of the laurel wreath, which was also awarded for victory in ancient Olympic games and continues to this day, for example, to winners of the Boston Marathon. Moreover, as an evergreen, the enduring nature of victory is symbolized. However, one must be careful not to "rest" on one's laurels.

***

Patient safety is (and always has been) a cornerstone of anesthesiology. With the American Society of Anesthesiologists' adoption of minimal monitoring standards,[8] the first medical specialty society to do so, a line in the sand was drawn acknowledging the primacy of patient safety, paving the way for a continuum of monitoring standards and medical simulation.[9-13]

Yet a narrow definition of safety has limited utility in the context of anesthesia or any medical practice. Although safety has been at the forefront of anesthetic practice for a very long time, there are some considerable compromises with always playing it safe. First of all, blind devotion to safety may promote hesitation and indecision as well as parochial thoughts. Second, when bold intervention is required, preoccupation with safety as avoidance of risk may inhibit the breadth and extent of such intervention. Finally, it may limit discovery, exploration and creativity – some of the maverick approaches that are daring, not uncommonly foolhardly and, occasionally, groundbreaking A careful balance has to be struck. Dire situations during an anesthetic demand second-by-second vigilance, and consistently altruistic (and occasionally, heroic) action, like the "Miracle on the Hudson".[‡] Microhypotheses of causation are often created in the operating room or in other aspects of acute or critical care and tested via interventions made in an uncertain and often "best educated guess" environment. Delivery from harm – *Soteria*, or salvation – is a laudable goal; it sometimes takes considerable daring to do so. The opposite of "harm," in this context, is "daring."

[‡] On January 15, 2009, US Airways Flight 1549, an Airbus A320-214, struck a flock of Canada geese just northeast of the George Washington Bridge and lost all engine power. Pilots Chesley Sullenberger and Jeffrey Skiles glided the plane to a ditching in the Hudson River and all 155 people aboard were rescued by nearby boats.

Those who are preoccupied with safety may not be truly free in their decisions about clinical care because in uncertain, dynamically evolving clinical situations like the operating room or intensive care unit, courage, bravery and daring – heroic actions – are just as necessary, and indeed integral to – safety.

***

The Ancient view of Heroes, however, was not our current view. While modern heroes often appear without fault – paragons – Hellenic Heroes were amplified in both their virtues as well as their sins. Heroes made mistakes and were held to account and punished by the gods. Some mortals, such as Herakles, were assigned seemingly impossible tasks, such as the Twelve Labors, in order to obtain redemption for the murder of his wife and children while temporarily insane. Akhilles, greatest of the Trojan warriors and slayer of Hector, the Trojan prince, died from Paris' arrow to his heel. Before that, notwithstanding his battle prowess, his pride, anger and cruelty in battle marked him for dishonor in war. Perseus was the slayer of the Medusa – then using the Medusa's head, turned Phineus (betrothed to Andromeda) to stone. They could be worshipped as heroes – or vilified when wrong! This dialectic offers a broader interpretation to "safety" because it incorporates courage, bravery and daring with risk and vulnerability.

Daring was an essential characteristic of Classical heroes and was vested in a specific, mortal personification. Heroes were mortal notwithstanding their descent from immortal gods. Because Heroes were god-like but mortal, they were vulnerable. That vulnerability made them understand that life was temporary and death inevitable, therefore, they understood and did not fear their own mortality. Similar superhuman feats and defeats befell Odysseus, Theseus and Jason. Bellerophon, having captured and tamed the wild stallion Pegasus, believed himself to have become a god and tried to ride to Mount Olympos, only to enrage Zeus to the point where Zeus made him fall to earth and die. The significance of their superhuman powers, in keeping with the Greek dialectic, was that they had superhuman faults as well. Their mortality implied that they performed their heroic feats without the loss of fear that immortality would have conferred – they had much more at stake than the gods.

The continuum of compassion, altruism and heroism can be included together in the concept of prosocial actions.[14] This social heroism is distinct from military (martial) or civic heroism and typically involves elements that are consistently seen in spontaneous and unconventional courageous professional interventions in the operating room and other medical care areas. That they do not involve immediate physical peril like martial heroism does not mean that risk is eliminated nor harsh judgement avoided for failure:[14]

1. There is an element of peril or sacrifice. While this is typically physical peril (for example, in military or fire rescue situations), in operating room interventions the perils are more related to the uncertainty of outcome or data on which to fully justify decisions. There is the risk of criticism based on inaccurately assessed situations or foolhardy actions.
2. The uncertain and rapidly evolving adverse situation is fraught with the fear and demand of acting decisively. Fear (*Phobos*) (see Chapter 12) is a major emotional challenge to be mastered in the crisis setting. The irony is that the presence of Strife (*Eris*) in the same setting may promote cognitive convergence (everyone thinking along the same lines) rather than its opposite, cognitive broadening. While this encourages focus, it may also limit breadth of thinking.

When viewed as a continuum, compassion, altruism and heroism represent a "heroic core" of prosocial values. More than just altruism as a professional value, is it reasonable to cultivate and develop a heroic core as a component of medical professionalism? Can an individual or a group cultivate a prime directive such as a "decision to act?" This has been described as the exquisite disparity between the public act of heroism versus the "interiority" of the decision to act in a heroic manner "which occurs before and in the absence of public knowledge about what is about to unfold."[14]

There are differences in the level of risk, velocity, and barriers to entry between altruism and heroism. However, the level of risk incurred in altruism is lower than even the minimum risk for heroism. How do we explain the disparity between "everyone *should* act, but not everyone *does* act?" Are there lessons to be learned from highly trained teams such as military special forces, tactical police teams and professional sports teams with regard to readying a mind-set for safety as well as heroism so that the initiation of critical action is favored at the earliest possible time? This is at the core, and part of the hidden curriculum, of medical simulation. There is a difference in the speed of the altruistic and heroic act. Deliberative indecision can occur from seconds to minutes in the altruistic act in increasingly ambiguous situations while heroic decisions tend to take place in a split-second, with actions that speedily move forward despite the complexity of the situation. Such situations seem more guided by mindfulness than by vigilance and concentration.[15]

Every person has the potential for developing their own continuum of prosocial actions, from safety through compassion, altruism and heroism. Anesthetists "dare" to impose unconsciousness, pain relief and complete dependence on medications, specialized skills, judgment, equipment and knowledge on those who enter the contract with uncertainty. When regarded as interlocking components of prosocial action, broader opportunities can be developed to prepare and then act in complex, uncertain situations. The general professionalism required of all anesthesiologists is mentioned in the Guidelines for the Ethical Practice of Anesthesiology.[16] Noteworthy is the distinction that "anesthetized patients are particularly vulnerable," i.e., the responsibility of the clinician is life support, breath by breath. While recklessness is to be condemned, the *pas de deux* of Safety and Daring – vigilant, circumspect, cautious as well as bold, fearless, and courageous – remain a delicate balance in the operating room, much of it the daily province of the anesthetist.

References

1. Kohn L, Corrigan J, Donaldson M. *To Err Is Human: Building a Safer Health System.* Washington, DC, National Academy Press, 2000.
2. Cooper J, Newbower R, Long C, McPeek B. Preventable anesthesia mishaps: a study of human factors. *Anesthesiology* 1978; 49: 399–406.
3. Thayer J. *The King James Version New Testament Greek Lexicon, Thayer and Smith's Bible Dictionary.* New York, NY, American Book Co, 1889.
4. Rosin H. *The Overprotected Kid*, The Atlantic, 2014.
5. Pausanias. *Description of Greece*, 7. 23. 9.
6. Pausanias. *Description of Greece*, 7. 19. 7.

7. Pausanias. *Description of Greece.* 7.21.7.
8. Eichhorn J, Cooper JB, Cullen D, Maier W, Philip J, Seeman R. Standards for patient monitoring during anesthesia at Harvard Medical School. *JAMA* 1986; 256: 1017–20.
9. Eichhorn J, Cooper JB, Cullen D, Gessner J, Holzman R, Maier W, Philip J. Anesthesia practice standards at Harvard: a review. *J Clin Anesth* 1988; 1: 55–65.
10. Cullen D, Eichhorn J, Cooper J, Maier W, Philip J, Holzman R, Gessner J. Postanesthesia care unit standards for anesthesiologists. *J of Post Anesthesia Nursing* 1989; 4: 141–6.
11. Cooper J, Cullen D, Eichhorn J, Philip J, Holzman R. Administrative guidelines for response to an adverse anesthesia event. *J Clin Anesth* 1993; 5: 79–84.
12. Holzman R, Cullen D, Eichhorn J, Philip J: Guidelines for sedation by nonanesthesiologists during diagnostic and therapeutic procedures. *J Clin Anesth* 1994; 6: 265–76.
13. Holzman R, Cooper J, Gaba D, Philip J, Small S, Feinstein D. Anesthesia crisis resource management: real-life simulation training in operating room crises. *J Clin Anesth* 1995; 7: 675–87.
14. Franco Z, Blau K, Zimbardo P. Heroism: a conceptual analysis and differentiation between heroic action and altruism. *Review of General Psychology* 2011; 15: 99–113.
15. Holzman R. Mindfulness and anesthesiology. *ASA Refresher Courses In Anesthesiology* 2014; 42: 75–82.
16. Committee on Ethics American Society of Anesthesiologists. *Guidelines for the Ethical Practice of Anesthesiology.* Park Ridge, IL, American Society of Anesthesiologists, 2013.

5

THE SPIRITS OF PAIN AND SUFFERING: THE *ALGEA*

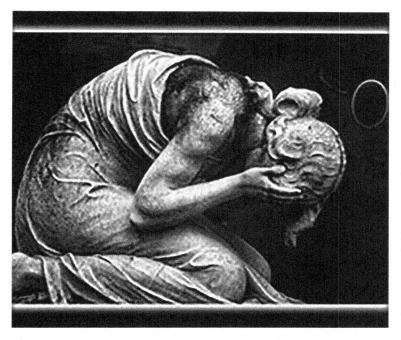

The *Algea* (L. *Dolores*) were the spirits of pain and suffering as well as grief, sorrow, and distress. Illustrated here as one goddess, there were three spirits described – *Lupe* (Lupa, L.), the spirit of pain, grief and distress, *Ania* (Ania, L.), the spirit of grief, distress, sorrow and trouble, and *Akhos* (Achos, L.), the spirit of ache and anguish.

Anesthesia is broadly considered to be the provision of pain relief, unconsciousness and motionlessness during surgery. Most surgical anesthetics are general anesthetics, but anesthetic techniques are much more extensive than that. They include

DOI: 10.1201/9781003201328-7

regional (nerve block) anesthesia, the provision of pain relief through the use of local anesthetic blocking major nerves to the arms or legs, as well as spinal or epidural anesthesia, blocking spinal nerves, typically for obstetrical pain relief or extremity surgery. Pain treatment specialists perform specific nerve blocks for the treatment of cancer pain, trauma, inflammatory diseases, headache and other disorders that can be treated with such blocks. They will also employ multi-modal analgesic medications because of their expert understanding of the various kinds of nerves and neurotransmitters involved in different modalities of pain – the lancinating pain of trauma, the sharp, twinging of peripheral neuropathies such as diabetic neuropathy, and the burning of complex regional pain syndromes. Critical Care Medicine, a melting pot of medical specialties such as anesthesiology, surgery, pulmonary medicine and pediatrics, began in the back of the Recovery Room (now called the Post Anesthesia Care Unit, or PACU) with anesthesiologists, as specialists in cardiopulmonary support and mechanical ventilation.

Pain is generally considered a symptom of an underlying condition, and medical approaches have traditionally focused on the underlying condition in order to treat the primary cause of the pain. As we now understand, pain itself causes suffering and alters an individual's neurobiology, independent of the underlying cause. The International Association for the Study of Pain begins its definition of pain with "*an unpleasant sensory and emotional experience* associated with actual or potential tissue damage ..."[1] which sets the stage for the complex physiological and emotional milieu within which pain occurs, propagates and endures.

Over the last several decades, the complex, intertwined relationship of pain, depression and the response to chronic inflammation has fueled the concept of the psychoneuroendocrine response to chronic pain, including a context for understanding the mutual contributions of each of these derangements to the other.[2] In addition, it provides an important model for the medical interventions that have proven successful as part of the treatment process[3] including the salutary role for selective serotonin and norepinephrine reuptake inhibitors in the management of depression. The influence of depression on pain as well as pain on depression is multidimensional and reciprocally amplifying and rectifying.

***

Pain in Homer's epics typically resulted from battle wounds, but by no means was the sufferer restricted to somatic pain. Far less emphasis was placed on the physical aspects in favor of concentrating on the more metaphysical, emotional and social accompaniments of physical pain. At least six groups of words were used to describe pain in Classical literature:[4]

Penthos: the pain of mourning
Kedos: grief, worry and obsession
Achos: worry and obsession, with despondency.
Odune: typically, a sharp, shooting pain, well localized, characterized as *oxus* or *pikros* (sharp and pointed or cutting and biting.) It was intended to reflect the weapon used to inflict the pain.
Pema: the suffix -ma denotes the personal involvement of the subject of the verb; the one who suffers through no fault of his own.
Algos: a more general type of suffering involving the whole body, vague in nature and undefined; cephalgia (headache) is a direct descendant. It implies prolonged suffering.

This provided an intriguing social context for pain, much more nuanced than anesthesiologists typically acknowledge in their daily work. Pain in association with combat truncated the breadth of the pain experience as we know it; pain associated with the immediacy of battle was acute pain, not the chronic pain of illness nor the suffering of persistent injury.

***

The *Algea* (L. Dolores) were the spirits of pain and suffering as well as grief, sorrow and distress. Their opposites were *Hedone*, the goddess of pleasure, and the *Kharites*, the goddesses of joy. The three *Algea* were *Lupe* (Lupa, L.), the spirit of pain, grief and distress, *Ania* (Ania, L.), the spirit of grief, distress, sorrow and trouble, and *Akhos* (Achos, L.), the spirit of ache and anguish.

Hesiod describes their genealogy and character only briefly:

> But abhorred *Eris* (Strife) bare painful *Ponos* (Toil), and *Lethe* (Forgetfulness), and *Limos* (Starvation), and the *Algea* (Pains), full of weeping ...[5]

but the Anacreonta[6] makes a prescient link between pain and its relief:

> Thanks to him (Dionysos), Methe (Drunkenness) was brought forth, the Kharis (Charis, Grace) was born, *Lupe (Pain) takes rest and Ania (Grief) goes to sleep.*
> (italics added)

once again, linking drug-induced sleep with relief from pain and suffering.

Few words conveyed pain as a physical experience; it was rather thought of as a metaphysical, perhaps existential experience, equivalent to misery, suffering, and in the psychological sense, grief, mourning, and loss (of existence). Superficially, it is not hard to picture this in the context of wounding as almost inevitable in a warring society. "Heroic" war injury was lauded, leaving the real suffering to be perceived as something metaphysical. Available soporifics like mandrake, hemp and opium addressed both.

Seneca metaphorically employed Oedipus to describe the scourge and the components of suffering as well as provide hope for relief:[7]

> After blinding himself and heading into exile, Oidipous (Oedipus) urges the pestilent daimones to leave Thebes:
> "All ye who are weary in body and burdened with disease, whose hearts are faint within you, see, I fly, I leave you; lift your heads.
> Milder skies come when I am gone. He who, though near to death, still keeps some feeble life, may freely now draw deep, life-giving draughts of air. Go, bear ye aid to those given up to death; all pestilential humours of the land I take with me.
> Ye blasting *Fatae* (Fates; *Keres*), thou quaking terror of *Morbus* (Disease, or *Nosos*), *Macies* (Wasting, or *Ischnasia*) and black *Pestis* (Pestilence, *Nosos*), and mad *Dolor*

(Despair, *Algos*), come ye with me, with me. Tis sweet to have such guides.²

The references to pain within the Hippocratic Collections are more focused; they have a tendency toward *odune*, the specific pain of injury, as opposed to *algos*, the more prolonged and vague suffering. The distinction, especially in the context of battle injuries, is that *odune* has a specific localization (which allowed prognostication, the highest form of Hippocratic medicine) whereas *algos* did not.

> In convalescents from diseases, if any part be pained, there deposits are formed.⁸
>
> (Aphorism 32)

In other Hippocratic works, *Ponos*, describing generalized suffering, is also used. The text *Of Art*, in describing a physician's duties, states that his job is to relieve *suffering*,⁹ a much broader challenge than somatic pain relief because it encompasses the whole person (see Chapter 19).

Therapeutic intervention is often represented in Hippocratic treatment by opposites, i.e., heat is treated with cold, dryness is treated with wetness, and in general, opposites cure opposites. In other instances, like could cure like, and this was the case for pain:

> Of two pains occurring together, not in the same part of the body, the stronger weakens the other.⁸
>
> (Aphorisms Section II, no. 46)

an observation heralding the gate control theory of pain* by more than two millennia.

***

Surgery as well as medical disease can lead to acute and chronic pain. In addition, the neurobiological effects of pain are such that they may result in the misery and suffering that accompany chronic pain. This sequence may very well be kindled by acute surgical pain, which is a principal focus of the perioperative experience. At the same time, the role of depression and other

---

* Non-painful sensations can override and reduce painful sensations.

psychiatric/emotional factors, well recognized in chronic pain management, are barely touched upon in current planning for surgical anesthesia or critical care, providing fertile ground for future efforts. It is astonishingly prescient that this connection was recognized by ancient avatars so long ago.

References

1. International Association for the Study of Pain (IASP) Task Force on Taxonomy, Part III. *Pain Terms, a Current List with Definitions and Notes on Usage*, Second Edition. Merskey H, Bogduk N (Eds). Seattle, WA, IASP Press, 1994, pp 209–14.
2. Leonard, B. Pain, depression and inflammation: are interconnected causative factors involved? *Mod Trends Pharmacopsychiatry* 2015; 30: 22–35.
3. Maletic V, Robinson M, Oakes T, Iyengar S, Ball S, Russell J. Neurobiology of depression: an integrated view of key findings. *Int J Clin Pract* 2007; 61: 2030–40.
4. Rey R. *The History of Pain*. Cambridge, MA, Harvard University Press. Translated by: Wallace L, Cadden J, Cadden S, 1995.
5. Hesiod. *Theogony*. Translated by: Evelyn-White, HG, l, 230 ff.
6. *The Anacreonta (Principal Remains of Anacreon of Teos Greek Lyric II*. London, JM Dent & Sons, Ltd. Translated by: Pope C, 1915.
7. Seneca. *Oedipus*, C 1st AD, l, 1052 ff.
8. Hippocrates. *Aphorisms, The Internet Classics Archive*, 400 BCE.
9. Hippocrates. *On the Art of Medicine*. Mann, JE (ed) Leiden, The Netherlands, Koninklijke Brill NV, 2012.

6
ANESTHESIA: "A NOT-FEELING PAIN"

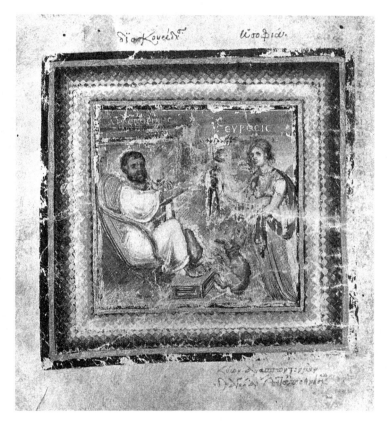

Dioscorides receives the mandrake from *Euresis*, the goddess of discovery. Immediately beneath the mandrake, a dog is rearing itself on its hindquarters, in *extremis* after the retrieval of the root (from the original in the Greek "Manuscript Anicia" of Dioscorides, in Venice, c. 512). (Unknown author, public domain, via Wikimedia Commons.)

DOI: 10.1201/9781003201328-8

Between October 16 and November 21, 1846, in the frenzied search for the right word for the recently demonstrated state of surgical insensibility, Dr. Oliver Wendell Holmes' proposal – "anaesthesia" – was "le mot juste" – *exactly* the correct word. His prophetic choice, however, had also been used in the recent as well as remote past, indeed, at the very beginning of recorded Classical civilization.

***

Hippocrates (460–380 BCE) may have been the first to use the word anesthesia to describe a (metaphysical) state by writing "The patient noticed nothing" ("anaisthesios") and "she took no notice of anything" ("anaisthesios").[1] This use seemed related more to cognition than sensation, but it was nevertheless important because it linked perception to sensation.

Theophrastus (380–287 BC), Alexander the Great's (356–323 BCE) classmate and fellow pupil of Aristotle (384–322 BCE) classified plants and noted their medicinal properties according to their *individual* characteristics rather than categorizing combinations of plants. This was a departure from traditional Egyptian formularies. He provided the earliest reference in Greek literature to mandragora, found in his *Enquiry into Plants*:

> The leaf of mandrake, they say, is useful for wounds, and the root for erysipelas,* when scraped and steeped in vinegar, and also for gout, *for sleeplessness* and for love potions.[2]
>
> (italics added, for emphasis)

Erasistratos (300–260 BCE), the physician to King Sleukos Nicator, gained fame after diagnosing the cause of the melancholy of Antiochus, the king's son, by monitoring the pulse of the young prince as the ladies of the court passed in front of him.†

---

* A relatively common bacterial infection of the superficial layer of the skin.
† While *Erasistratos* was examining the patient, *Stratonice*, one of the elderly king's wives, entered the room. From the increase in the young prince's pulse and from the flush that spread over his cheeks, *Erasistratos* recognized that the illness was mental rather than physical – that a passion for his inaccessible stepmother was the etiology of the trouble. Of course, an increase in pulse rate and facial flushing are well-recognized side effects of belladonna alkaloids.

His pulse quickened as his stepmother passed in front of him. Misleading as this might have been given mandrake's anticholinergic and aphrodisiac properties, Erasistratos, by palpating the pulse continuously, diagnosed the case as love, and persuaded the king to divorce his wife and let his son marry her.[3] Consolidation and codification of medicinals was provided in the 1st century CE by Dioscorides, Nero's surgeon, who collected all the information he could on drugs and published his *Materia Medica*. This was a logical extension of the efforts of Theophrastus because each drug was discussed according to its various names, sources, and means of identification, risks of adulteration, method of preparation as well as indication. In this manner, Dioscorides described some 600 plants and non-plant materials, including metals.[3] His description of mandragora is famous – the root of which he indicates may be made into a preparation that will cause some degree of sleepiness and relief of pain:

> And some do seethe the roots in wine to thirds, and straining it set it up. Using a Cyathus ‡ of it for such as cannot sleep, or are grievously pained, and upon whom being cut, or cauterized they wish to make *a not-feeling pain*. Ye juice being drank ye muchness of ye quantity of 2 Oboli§ with Melicrate,** doth expel upward Phlegm, and black choler, as Eleebore†† doth, but being too much drank it drives out ye life ... and being put up into ye seat for a suppository, it causeth sleep. Ye wine of ye bark of ye root is prepared without seething but you must cast in 3 pounds into a Metreta‡‡ of sweet wine, and that there be given of it 3 Cyathi to such as shall be cut,

---

‡ In ancient Greece, the cyathus was a wine ladle, used as a server from a larger vessel; its liquid measure was equal to one twelfth of a sextarius, approximately 42 ml or 1.5 oz.
§ An ancient Greek coin or weight equal to one sixth of a drachma. From the Latin obolus and Greek obolos (obelos), literally, "spit," which also meant nail. Nails were used as money, with six of them making a handful (drachme).
** A fermented or unfermented beverage of honey and water
†† Form of Hellebore, a poisonous herb of the genus helleborus or veratrum, containing alkaloids that may have been used variously as cardiac and respiratory depressant agents.
‡‡ An ancient Greek liquid measure, equivalent to approximately nine gallons.

or cauterized, as is aforesaid. For they do not apprehend the pain, because they are overborn with dead sleep ... but used too much they make men speechless ... Physitians also, use this, when they are about to cut, or cauterize.[3]

In his description of mandragora, Dioscorides uses the word anesthesia ("a not-feeling pain") for the first time in a non-cognitive sense. He emphasized that when physicians are about to cut or burn a patient they should give him mandrake wine to cause insensibility. There is a subtle, but critical difference – the Greek "anaisthesia" (αναισθησια-insensibility) is from a- (without) + aisthesis (perception), as distinct from "anodyne" (ανοδυνη), a pain-relieving remedy, derived from a- (without) + odune (pain). This was different from its apparent prior use by Hippocrates. There were actually many names for pain in the ancient world (*vide supra*); had any of them caught on, it is likely we might not now be known as anesthesiologists but rather as *algologists* (Greek) or *dolorologists* (Latin).

Scribonius Largus, also in the 1st century, compiled *Compositiones Medicorum* and gave the first description of opium in Western medicine, describing the way by which the juice issues from the unripe seed capsule and how it is gathered after it is dried for use. It was suggested by the author that it be given in a water emulsion for the purpose of producing sleep and relieving pain.[4] Galen (129–199 CE), another Greek, studied anatomy and medicine for 12 years at Pergamon, Smyrna, Corinth and Alexandria, worked as a surgeon in the gladiatorial school at Pergamon and then practiced as a physician, surgeon and druggist in Rome. His *De Simplicibus* (about 180 AD) was the only Greek herbal comparable to that of Dioscorides and described plant, animal and mineral materials in a systematic and rational manner. It also became a major reference source for centuries afterward. His prescriptions suggested rational use for opium and hyoscyamus, among others, and while his formulations became known as *galenicals*, the word anesthesia was not used in conjunction with their administration.

Knowledge of herbs and medicinals during the Dark Ages (5th to 11th centuries) was maintained through the efforts of scribes in Constantinople (the capitol of the Eastern Roman Empire) and then in the Muslim Empire. Health professions all but vanished within the jurisdiction of the Church and drug use returned to primitive empiricism, magic and witchcraft. Western monks acquired simple medical skills, but religious healers and secular medical craftsmen did not always work together harmoniously.

The first Christian medieval reference to what we recognize as anesthesia, unconsciousness and pain relief for surgery is found in the 4th century in the writings of Hilary (c. 310–367 CE), the bishop of Poitiers. In his treatise on the Trinity, Hilary distinguished between anesthesia or loss of sensation due to disease and intentional anesthesia resulting from drugs, walking a careful line between scholarship and heresy:

> The nature of our bodies is such, that when imbued with life and feeling *by conjunction with a sentient soul,* they become something more than inert, insensate matter. They *feel* when touched, *suffer* when pricked, *shiver* with cold, *feel pleasure* in warmth, *waste* with hunger and *grow fat* with food ... For instance a flesh wound is felt even to the bone, while the fingers feel nothing when we cut the nails, which protrude from the flesh ... Also when through some grave necessity part of the body must be cut away, *the soul can be lulled to sleep by drugs, which overcome the pain and produce in the mind a death-like forgetfulness of its power of sense.* Then limbs can be cut off without pain.[5]

This fusion of body and soul in the context of Church doctrine conferred an ecclesiastical legitimacy to neurophysiology and pharmacology. While St. Hilary does not describe the drugs that lulled the soul to sleep, at this time (and for the following few centuries) the emphasis remained on mandragora.

Pseudo-Apuleius, a 4th century compiler of Greek botanico-medical material, recognized the importance of the therapeutic index of such potent drugs:

> If any one eat it he will die immediately unless he be treated with butter and honey, and vomit quickly. Further, if any one is to have a limb mutilated, burnt, or sawn, he may drink half an ounce with wine, and whilst he sleeps the member may be cut off without any pain or sense.[6]

From 500 to 1400 CE the Church greatly expanded its empire and clearly was the dominant institution in all walks of life. The Church controlled scholarship, or what passed for scholarship, which was primarily hand copying of valued, ancient Greek and Roman manuscripts. Medical knowledge and healing activity tended to reside within ecclesiastical communities. However, monks did not copy or read medical books merely as an academic exercise; *Cassiodorus*, in an influential work on studies appropriate for monks, recommended books by Hippocrates, Galen and Dioscorides while linking the purpose of medical reading with charity care and help. Most of the advances of medicine began as extensions of Greco Roman and Muslim knowledge, greatly aided by trade and by the available information on plant and medicinal lore. The herbal of Dioscorides was blindly accepted as the authoritative source on medical plants for virtually the entire 1000-year interregnum of the Dark Ages. Eventually, Church Councils (1131–1212) prohibited monks from participating in medical practices; nevertheless, their libraries became the repositories of herbal knowledge and some monks left the cloister in order to pursue medical studies or practice medicine elsewhere. The Council of Clermont (1130) forbade the practice of medicine by the monks, and the Council of Tours, in 1163, declared the doctrine of "Ecclesia abhorret a sanguine" ("the Church does not shed blood").

By the middle years of the 12th century, the process that provided western European medicine with a rich, specialized literature, renowned centers of learning and a flourishing tradition of practice, was already well advanced. Various medical and drug compendia were translated from Greek and Arabic into Latin, beginning with *Constantinus Africanus* (1015–1087). His work was seminal; much effort was subsequently devoted into translating into Latin some of the Greco-Roman and Arab classics that continued to enter Europe during and following the Crusades. The rise of Universities at Paris (1110), Bologna (1113) Oxford (1167) and Montpelier (1181) may be related to this pattern. The foundational groundwork for late medieval and Renaissance medical culture had already been established.

Salerno

Conventional Greco-Roman drug tradition, organized and preserved by the Muslims, returned to Europe chiefly through Salerno, an important trade center on the southwest coast of Italy in the mid-900s. In the 10th century, local monastic medicine began to decline as a result of monks spending more time in medical pursuits and less time fulfilling their religious duties. Even in monastic circles, medical studies, medical practice and reliance on medicine were taking on a more secular and specialized cadre. Perhaps those who cared for the sick asked for more extensive reference works to help in their effort, which were no problem to obtain along the trade routes. Salerno evolved into a school of medicine, *remaining independent of Church regulation*. At the same time, cities were growing larger and secular universities were proliferating, events mirroring the growth of lay medicine. Salerno's medical melting pot was a hub of knowledge derived from sources as diverse as the ancient Greco Roman tradition (still present in southern Italy at the time), monastic medicine, and Jewish, Muslim and Oriental practices of the Far and Middle East and Northern Africa. Furthermore, by decree of Frederic II, the Holy Roman Emperor, only the Salernitan school was granted the right to license physicians to practice medicine. The combination of allowing surgery at a time when it was not considered a branch of medicine but merely a crude offshoot activity with no scientific basis plus herbals for pain relief in the absence of Church regulation, all the while flourishing as a crossroads of trade in a geographically central area made it almost inevitable that a center of medical learning would inevitably arise at Salerno! Surgery in Salerno, therefore, became a doctor's occupation, and not something simply entrusted to barbers and butchers. It was because of this secular view that surgery could include concepts of pain relief and unconsciousness that were not opposed by the Church.[7]

Singularly important in the history of pain relief at Salerno was intentional surgical anesthesia. *Practica Chirugiae*, written in 1170 by the surgeon Roger Frugardi (Roger of Salerno) mentions a sponge soaked in "narcotics" and held to the patient's nose. Hugh of Lucca (ca. 1160–1252) prepared such a sleeping sponge according to a prescription later described by Theodoric of Cervia (ca. 1205–1296):

> Take of opium, of the juice of the unripe mulberry, of hyoscyamus, of the juice of hemlock, of the juice of the leaves of mandragora, of the juice of the wood-ivy, of the juice of the forest mulberry, of the seeds of lettuce, of the seeds of the dock, which has large round apples, and of the water hemlock – each an ounce; mix all these in a brazen vessel, and then place in it a new sponge; let the whole boil, as long as the sun lasts on the dog-days, until the sponge consumes it all, and it is boiled away in it. As oft as there shall be need of it, place this sponge in hot water for an hour, and let it be applied to the nostrils of him who is to be operated on, until he has fallen asleep, and so let the surgery be performed. This being finished, in order to awaken him, apply another sponge, dipped in vinegar, frequently to the nose, or throw the juice of the root of fenugreek into the nostrils; shortly he awakes.

As an added precaution, however, Theodoric bound his patients prior to incision.

The description of the soporific sponge of Theodoric survived through the Renaissance largely because of Guy de Chauliac's (1300–1367) *The Grand Surgery* and the clinical practices of Hans von Gersdorff (c. 1519) and Giambattista della Porta (1535–1615), who used essentially the same formula. The herbalist William Turner (1510–1568) described the "forgetful and sleepish drowsiness" following the ingestion of a potion containing mandragora root as well as the pragmatic warning "they that smell too much of the apples, become dumb."[8]

The Age of Enlightenment

"Anaesthesia" once again appeared in Castelli's *Lexicon Medicum Graeco Latinum* (1665),[7] where it was subsequently translated as a "privation of the senses."[9] This may not have meant anything different than the cognitive privation referred to centuries earlier by Hippocrates. In 1718, "anaesthesia" was used by J.B. Quistorp (Quistorpius) (1692–1761) in a Latin philosophical dissertation

"De Anaesthesia" ("Anaesthesia, a state of insensitivity"). The thesis spoke about anesthesia in a metaphysical sense, lacking any further somatic detail. This thesis has been translated into English only recently. "Anaesthesia" first appeared in English in Bailey's Dictionary as "a loss or Defect of Sense, as in such as have the Palsy."[9] In 1819, Parr's Medical Dictionary defined anaesthesia as "insensibility or loss of feeling, by touch." [11] In 1845, McPheeters used "partial anaesthesia" to describe a loss of sensation below the knee without motor loss.[11]

The Public Demonstration of Ether

In 1846, William T.G. Morton was asked to demonstrate "the preparation you have invented to *diminish the sensibility to pain*" at the Ether Dome at Massachusetts General Hospital. After the demonstration, Dr. Jacob Bigelow of Harvard Medical School wrote to Dr. Francis Boott in London about "a new **anodyne** process."[13] Quickly realizing the historical moment and having observed firsthand his daughter's tooth extraction with a general anesthetic, Harvard's President Edward Everett wrote at least 12 different people in Britain about surgery with ether.[13] As Vice President of the American Academy of Arts and Sciences, Everett was present to hear Henry Jacob Bigelow deliver his first abstract on ether anesthesia. On November 14, the earliest of the Everett letters described "a *narcotic* gas to facilitate ... surgical operations." Everett also wrote on November 28 of "a method of producing a temporary *suspension of sensibility* by inhaling euphoric ether." On November 30, the prolific Everett wrote to Reverend Dr. Whewell, the Master of Trinity College, Cambridge, conveying a similar message. Writing to Dr. Francis Boott, Everett enclosed a copy of his November 4 address at the opening of Boston's new Medical College, having added a postscript following the delivery of the address, declaring "great confidence ... in inducing complete *insensibility* under the most cruel operations."[14]

Despite Dr. Oliver Wendell Holmes' 1886 neologism claim for "anaesthesia," his own letter to Morton 40 years earlier refers to prior use of the term to denote insensibility. The prevalent description "insensibility" suggested the term anesthesia rather than anodynia; the new process was not only a means of pain relief but also a means of unconsciousness and forgetfulness, a greater goal than simply pain relief. Some movement could be tolerated and various depths of anesthesia appreciated as long as the patient wouldn't remember (and presumably the operation could continue)!

***

Why a paean to anesthesia in the midst of a Pantheon of avatars of professional development? The specialty itself represents the poignancy of a search lasting millennia punctuated by a discovery a little over 150 years ago. The exponential growth in anesthesiology and its contributions to pharmacology, physiology, biochemistry, biomedical engineering, complex reasoning, to name just a few, now extend beyond these fields – to resuscitation, to advanced pulmonary care in the chronic care / rehabilitation setting and pain management in everyday life. How do "anesthesiologists" prepare themselves to succeed in these relatively new arenas while honoring the core of professional values? We are used to thinking of our specialty as a little over 150 years old, having celebrated the sesquicentennial just recently, yet history shows that the search for a terse label for the insensibility to pain as well as its metaphysical and philosophical implications – control, uncertainty, safety, daring, and the challenges of accumulating the requisite knowledge, judgment and wisdom – is as old as civilization and medical practice itself.

References

1. Hippocrates. *Case XV in Epidemics III, De morbis populairibus.* Edited by Jones W. Cambridge, Harvard University Press, 1868, line 285.
2. Pedanius Dioscorides of Anazarbos. *The Greek Herbal of Dioscorides, Illustrated by a Byzantine A.D. 512, Englished by John Goodyer A.D. 1655, Book 4.* Oxford, Oxford University Press. Translated by: Goodyer J, 1933.
3. Rey R. *The History of Pain.* Cambridge, Harvard University Press. Translated by: Wallace L, Cadden J, Cadden S, 1995.
4. Leake C. *An Historical Account of Pharmacology to the 20th Century*, Publ. No. 970. Springfield, IL, Charles C. Thomas, 1975.
5. St. Hilary of Poitiers. *The Trinity.* Baltimore, Catholic University of America Press. Translated by: McKenna S, 2002.

6. de Lignamine P. *The Herbal of Pseudo-Apuleius, from the Ninth-Century Manuscript in the Abbey of Monte Cassino (Codex Casinensis 97, Edition Princeps Romae 1481* Edited by Hunger F. Leyden, The Netherlands, Brill, 1481.
7. Castelli B. *Lexicon Medicum Graeco-Latinum Rotterdam, Apud Arnoldum Leers 1665*. Archives & Special Collections; Dickinson College; Carlisle, PA; archives@dickinson.edu.
8. Miller A. The origin of the word anaesthesia. *Boston Med Surg J* 1927: 1218–22.
9. Bailey N. *Dictionarium Britannicum*. London, T. Cox, 1730.
10. Parr B. *The London Medical Dictionary*. London, J. Johnson et al., 1809.
11. McPheeters W. Case of partial anaesthesia, with remarks. *Boston Med Surg J* 1845: 153–4.
12. Bigelow H. Insensibility during surgical operations produced by inhalation. *Boston Med Surg J* 1846; 35: 309–317.
13. Everett E. *Edward Everett Papers*. Boston, Massachusetts Historical Society, 1846.
14. Everett E. *Address delivered at the opening of the new Medical College in North Grove Street*, Boston, William Ticknor and Co, 1846.

Part II

QUALITIES

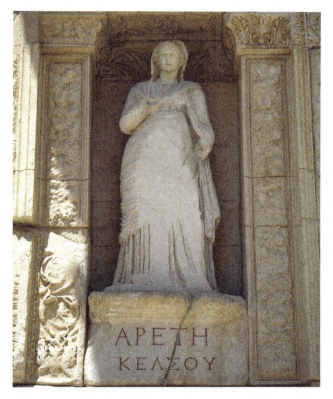

Arete was the goddess of virtue, excellence, goodness and valor. Personification of Virtue (Arete), the second statue from the façade of the Celsus library, in Ephesus, near Selçuk, west Turkey (second century).

DOI: 10.1201/9781003201328-9

There is a story that Virtue dwells on rocks which are hard to climb, (...) looks after the holy ground. She is not visible to the eyes of all mortal men, but only to him whose heart-eating sweat comes from within, the one who attains the peak of manliness.*

***

How then, does one become effective at understanding and treating the variations in the human condition? What qualities must be cultivated for coping with the uncertainties? Preparation and training, as for any endeavor – but what *enduring* qualities are required?

Certainly *Scholarship*, as embodied by *Kheiron* the Centaur, teacher of *Asklepios* and *Akhilles* (among many others) and the first medical educator. In addition, *Skill* is necessary, represented by *Tekhne*, the spirit of art, technical skill and craft, inseparable from *Hephaistos* (Vulcan) and the *Muses*. Moving beyond the concept of competencies into the current realms of milestones and entrustable professional activities, something more is desirable – independent mastery of beauty and articulation in craft and in thought, integral to the highest standards of practice across all specialties. *Beauty* and *Grace* embody the highest technical performance levels for any specialty, and include the ability to be articulate with colleagues and patients in the spoken and written word. Even these lofty achievements are the penultimate step. *Wisdom*, the ultimate step, personified by *Sophia*, crowns the previous values as the quintessential quality of professional development needed for the legitimate advancement of clinical practice.

What enduring virtues are required? There were numerous important dimensions to virtue for the ancient Greeks, beginning with the notion of fulfillment and living up to one's potential – being the best you can be. Unlike the literal gender reference of the above quote, *Virtue* was not gender specific. Homer applied the concept without regard to gender, and while bravery was a frequent associated value, effectiveness was an equal interpretation. At a higher level, Aristotle favored contemplation – knowledge

---

* Simonides, Fragment 579, cited in Demos, M. *Lyric Quotations in Plato.* Lanham, MD, Rowman and Littlefield, 1999, p. 15.

about knowledge – or epistemology. This concept was also at the core of Platonic and Socratic philosophy. Cultivating these essential qualities without hubris is a challenge for high-achieving professionals. In classical Greek tragedy, hubris was often a fatal shortcoming that brought about the fall of the tragic hero, regardless of the heroic achievements preceding the fall. Overconfidence led the hero to overstep the boundaries of human limitations and presume a godlike status. The gods inevitably humbled the offender with a sharp reminder of his or her mortality.

7
SCHOLARSHIP: *KHEIRON*

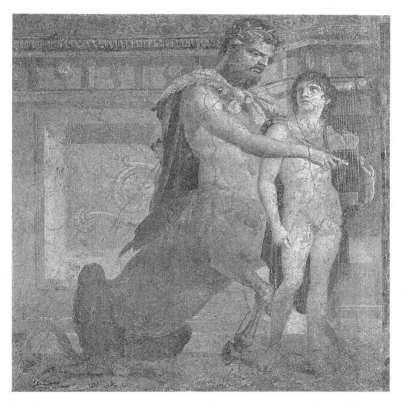

Kheiron instructs the young Akhilles.

The fresco shows the centaur *Kheiron*, Akhilles' pedagogue, teaching the young hero the use of the lyre. Roman fresco, National Archaeological Museum, Naples, Italy. (Sconosciuto Il prototipo era probabilmente un gruppo scultoreo esposto a Roma nei Saepta., public domain, via Wikimedia Commons.)

Prince Akhilles, suppliant to the towering, master Centaur, regarding him with a mixture of awe, fear and a suggestion of resentment. The Centaur's intensity is portrayed against the ominous backdrop of uncertainty, while the supplicant's naiveté is pale in comparison.

***

Educational achievement is a starter criterion for medical school and accomplishment in postgraduate medical education. One does well on Scholastic Achievement Tests (SATs) in order to enter the best college possible, Medical College Admissions Tests (MCATs) in order to enter the best medical school possible, passes National Board of Medical Examiner (NBME) exams, specialty exams, subspecialty exams to obtain board certification and so forth. Content-based knowledge is a justifiably large component of traditional medical education and practice. More recently, emphasis has been placed on the philosophy and resources necessary for continuing medical education, maintenance of certification and life-long learning, all of which are based on core principles of a continuing engagement with educational growth and development. It is, however, relatively easy in our current system of compliance with such goals to achieve benchmarks of credible public competency – having your college and medical school diploma, various subsequent postgraduate medical education certifications, and verification of acceptable credit for participation in continuing medical education. What is subtler is to continually challenge oneself with professional growth into evolving areas of uncertainty because they confront one's sensibilities of finitude and completion. In this context, the role of the medical educator expands to educator-motivator as well as role model.

***

Kheiron was the first medical educator in western civilization. He was the most senior and well known of the centaurs, the son of Kronos, renowned for wisdom and skill in medicine. He was the teacher and mentor of many heroes. His role as a medical educator, however, was emphasized in connection with the teaching of surgical skill and herbal lore to Asklepios and Akhilles, as well as other student-disciples.

Akhilles	The son of Peleus. When Akhilles' mother Thetis left home and returned to the Nereids,§ Peleus brought his son Akhilles to *Kheiron*, who received him as a disciple, and fed him the innards of lions and wild swine and the marrow of she-wolves.
Aktaeon	Aktaeon, bred by *Kheiron* to be a hunter, is famous for his terrible death. He was devoured by his own dogs after being turned into a deer for accidentally stumbling upon Artemis bathing. The dogs, ignorant of what they had done, came to the cave of *Kheiron* seeking their master, and the Centaur fashioned an image of Aktaeon in order to soothe their grief.
Ajax	A Greek hero who fought in the Trojan War. He is the son of Telamon, brother of Peleus.
Aristaeus	The Muses taught Aristaeus the arts of healing and of prophecy. Aristaeus discovered honey and the olive.
Asklepius	The great healing power of Asklepius is based on *Kheiron*'s teaching. Artemis killed Asklepius' mother Koronis on Apollo's orders while still pregnant after she had an affair. He snatched the child from the pyre and brought him to *Kheiron*, who reared him and taught him the arts of healing and hunting.
Herakles	The son of Zeus. Some versions of Greek mythology state that Herakles was trained by *Kheiron*.
Jason	In an early tradition, Aeson gave his son Jason to the Centaur *Kheiron* to rear at the time when he was deposed by King Pelias. Jason was the captain of the Argonauts.
Oileus	A member of the Argonauts.
Phoenix	A Myrmidon** who accompanied Akhilles in the Trojan War. *Kheiron* was the one who restored Phoenix's eyesight.
Patroklus	Patroklus' father, Menoetius, left him in *Kheiron*'s cave to study (side by side with Akhilles) the chords of the harp, learn to hurl spears and mount and ride upon the back of *Kheiron*.

---

§ Nereids are sea nymphs, particularly associated with the Aegean Sea.
** The Myrmidons were the mythological natives of Thessaly. During the Trojan War, they were commanded by Akhilles.

Peleus	Peleus, father of Akhilles, was once rescued by *Kheiron*, who subsequently arranged the marriage of Peleus with Thetis. He told Peleus how to conquer the Nereid Thetis who, changing her form, could prevent him from catching her.
Perseus	The son of Zeus. A Greek hero who was known for beheading Medusa.
Telamon	A Greek king father of Ajax and his half-brother Teucer.
Theseus	The son of king Aegeas of Athens. Known for slaying the Minotaur.

His name comes from *kheir*, the Greek word for hand, which, in a broader sense, meant "skilled with the hands." It was also associated with *kheirourgos*, (chirurgus (L)) or surgeon and there are numerous Classical references to his singular talents:

> When *Saturn* (Kronos, Gr.) was hunting *Jove* (Jupiter) throughout the earth, assuming the form of a steed, he lay with Philyra, daughter of Ocean (Oceanus). By him she bore Chiron the Centaur, who is said to have been the first to invent the art of healing.[1]

> Chiron, son of Saturn, first used herbs in the medical art of surgery; Apollo first practiced the art of treating eyes, and third, Asclepius, son of Apollo, began the art of clinical medicine.[2]

Even Pliny the Elder, among the many harsh Classical critics of physicians, referred to *Kheiron* with respect:

> The science of herbs and drugs was discovered by Chiron the son of Saturnus (Kronos) and Philyra.[3]

Of particular interest for anesthesia was *Kheiron*'s singular teaching role with regard to pain management. For pain resulting from battle injury, the most common cause of pain in recorded Greek medicine, Eurypylos addressed Patroklos during the Trojan War, according to Homer:

Cut the arrow out of my thigh ... and put kind medicines on it, good ones, which they say you have been told of by Akhilleus, since Kheiron, most righteous of the Kentauroi, told him about them.[4]

A specific herbal, for the most part mandrake, was employed by the Ancients for pain relief, with careful invocation of *Kheiron*'s approval:

> What ridge of the pasturing woodlands must I traverse to summon old lifebringing *Kheiron* to help your wound? Or where can I find medicines, the secrets of Paieon the Healer's (Asklepios) pain-assuaging art? Would that I had what they call the herb *Kentaurida* (of the Centaur), that I might bind *the flower of no-pain* (italics added) upon your limbs, and bring you back safe and living from Haides whence none returns! What magic hymn have I, or song from the stars, that I may chant the ditty with Euian voice divine, and stay the flow of blood from your wounded side? Would I had here beside me the fountain of life, that I might pour on your limbs that painstilling water and assuage your adorable wound, to bring back even your soul to you again![5]

Kheiron's prowess in the practice of pain relief, a large share of his practice in a warring society, was merely a part of his responsibility. Of greater importance, the notion of education consignment – *the placement of a student in the hands of an expert educator who has special knowledge to impart* – was a seismic change from education within the family to the family tradition or trade. Prince Akhilles was removed from the family setting, in fact, from all family, to obtain instruction from a teacher who is so far removed that he was a different species! Yet he possessed the knowledge, skill and qualities of character that make him ideal – a noble schoolmaster.

Syr Thomas Eliot (1538) described the breadth of *Kheiron*'s pedagogy:

> Chiron, nis,[*] the name of a man, whom poetes doo fayne to be the one halfe of a man, the other halfe lyke a hors:

---

[*] Old English contraction, from ne is ("is not").

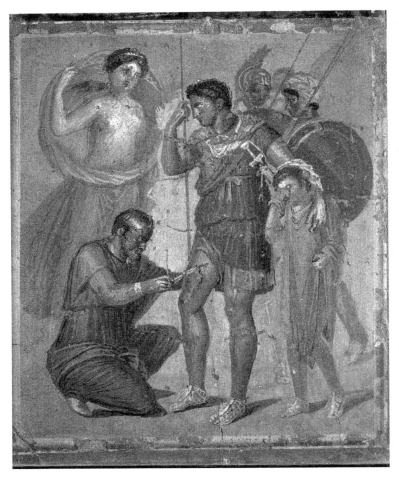

The Fresco of Iapyx. Ascanius weeps beside his wounded father, Aeneas, who is supporting himself with a lance in his right hand. Close by, shrouded in mist, Aeneas' divine mother, Aphrodite, descends from heaven, while the Greek surgeon, Iapyx, pulls out the arrowhead with his forceps. (Élisée Reclus, public domain, via Wikimedia Commons.)

who fyrst dyd fynde the vertues of herbes, and taughte Aesculapius phisike, and Apollo to harpe, and Astronomy to Hercules, and was mater to Achylles, and excelled all other men of his tyme in vertue and iustyce.[6]

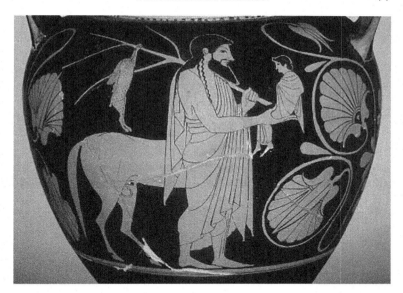

The centaur *Kheiron* holds the boy Akhilles in one hand and in the other a branch with a hanging hare. The centaur is depicted with the full body of a man – including legs and feet – with the torso and rear legs of a horse. (Collection of Giampietro Campana di Cavelli; 1861. Musée du Louvre.)

Artistic representations of *Kheiron* were initially painted on ceramic vessels of the seventh and 6th centuries BCE. His human half was sober, erect, dignified, with impeccable grooming, befitting the most senior of the centaurs. He was often shown with Akhilles, receiving him as an infant from the hands of Peleus, the father of Akhilles.

Why leave an infant in the care of a centaur? Not surprisingly, Machiavelli offered some interesting thoughts on this question:

> You must know that there are two ways of contesting, the one by law, the other by force; the first method is proper to men, the second to beasts; but because the first is frequently not sufficient, it is necessary to have recourse to the second. Therefore *it is necessary for a prince to understand how*

to avail himself of the beast and the man. This has been figuratively taught to princes by ancient writers who describe how Achilles and many other princes of old were given to the centaur Chiron to raise, who brought them up in his discipline; which means solely that, as they had for a teacher one who was half beast and half man, so *it is necessary for a prince to know how to make use of both natures, and that the one without the other is not durable.*[7]

Machiavelli's vision was that the centaur symbolized dualities in nature, society and education. The goal of education was to make the prince both wise as well as powerful. Erasmus expressed the idea as well: "Chiron taught his pupils to play the lyre, but he taught them also the fierceness of centaurs."

Kheiron's Dialectic of Scholarship and Brutality

Kheiron was isolated physically as well as metaphysically from the rest of the centaurs. This isolation allowed focus on the educator/mentor himself, a somewhat charlatanic turn for the otherwise noble but humble *Kheiron*. His physical appearance declared his status and heritage. His front legs were often described or portrayed as human rather than equine, especially in early works of art, in contrast to the traditional representation of centaurs, which have the entire lower body of a horse.[8] This further set *Kheiron* apart from the other centaurs, making him easily identifiable. Behaviorally, the centaurs were said to lead a wild and savage life in Thessaly and were fond of rowdy celebrations. They came to symbolize dark and unruly forces of nature, proxies for the blind and brute force of human nature.

Yet his brutal side was not denied, rather controlled. A seventeenth-century illustration showed *Kheiron* with the motto "Exercet Utrumque" ("He practices both"). The unclothed centaur holds a club over his right shoulder and an open book in his left hand. Behind him is a body of water, a castle at its edge, and high hills in the background. In another reference,[9] it is captioned "Pour l'un et l"autre" ("for the one and the other"), with the following French inscription:

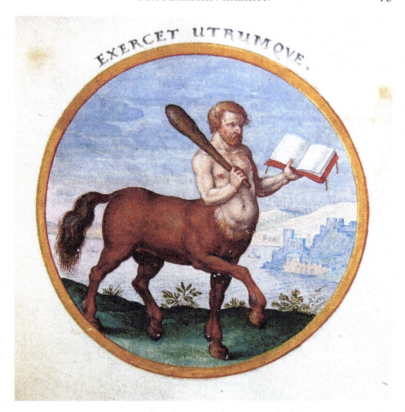

Gloria Crocodilus / Exercet utrumque. From an album of 82 leaves by Jacob Hoefnagel, 1634. (British Museum; Museum number 1994, 1001.10.28.)

> Le livre d'une main la massue de lautre,
> Cettecy est du corps, cestuila de lesprit
> Chiron par son exemple a son Achille apprit,
> Que pour bien vivre il faut exercer l'un et l'autre.†

With the depiction of the dialectic – the book in one hand, the club in the other, this of the body, that of the mind – *Kheiron*, by

---

† The book in one hand and the club in the other,
  This is for the body, this is for the mind
  Chiron by his example to his Achilles taught,
  That to live well you have to exercise both.

his own example, taught Akhilles that to live well it was necessary to exercise both (i.e. "the one and the other").

A further moral is implied by the fusion; as a result of the conflict between these powerful drives, to maintain themselves as human, the centaur must not allow his base appetites to overcome integrity, lest he indeed becomes an "'hommecheval' devoid of true wisdom."[10] Machiavelli recognized this problem well in describing the political facts of life, a recurring theme in ancient and contemporary culture. (see section VII)

The Brutal *Kheiron*: The Achilleid and Polycraticus

John of Salisbury (1115/20–1180) wrote the Polycraticus (1159), portraying the brutal side of *Kheiron*, describing his curriculum

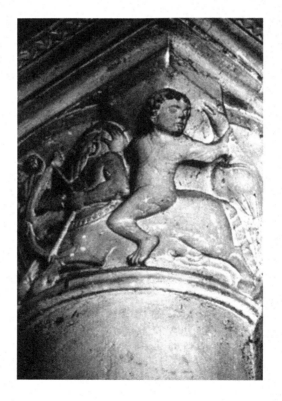

Kheiron and Akhilles hunting lesson. Column capital, Chartres Cathedral. (Courtesy of J. Jacobson, University of Minnesota, The College of Education and Human Development.)

of blood, killing, and endurance testing; the sculpture of *Kheiron* and Akhilles in the Chartres Cathedral is in keeping with that tradition. On a column capital just inside the Royal Portal, a centaur, armed with bow and arrow, supports Akhilles on his back while the boy appears to strangle a large bird.

Serendipity may have played a role here – the sculpture was probably carved while John was a student at the Cathedral school between 1137 and 1140. He certainly would have seen it when he returned as Archbishop in 1176. In his writings he interprets the half-beast desires cultivated by *Kheiron* to act against the elements of humanity and delivers an invective against the blood sports of kings and courtiers:

> To this day, hunters smack of the Centaurs' training. Rarely is one found to be modest or dignified, rarely self-controlled, and in my opinion never temperate. They were indeed imbued with these characteristics in the home of Chiron.[11]

He advocates for practical reason and self-discipline dominating over appetite; he controls the horse beneath his head and heart, the discipline of self-judgment over impulse. These ethical precepts contain the rudiments of moral philosophy essential to a social life and transcend barbarism. Allegorically, they also provide guidance for comportment during the "blood sport" of the operating room, particularly for conflict resolution. The urging of modesty, dignity, self-control and temperance thus become cornerstones of professional civility.

The Death of *Kheiron*

The master teacher's ultimate lesson occurred with his final exit. As the son of Kronos, a Titan, *Kheiron* was immortal. Yet the impossible occurs; he does indeed die.

It was left to Herakles to arrange a deal with Zeus to exchange *Kheiron*'s immortality for the life of Prometheus, chained to a rock and left to die for stealing fire from Mt. Olympos and giving fire to man. *Kheiron* was accidentally poisoned with an arrow belonging to Herakles that had been treated with the blood of the Hydra.‡ The wound was incurable and unbearably painful.

---

‡ A serpentine water monster with poisonous breath and blood so virulent that even its scent was deadly.

Kheiron voluntarily relinquished his immortality and died to free himself from the pain. Instead of going to Haides, he was given a place amongst the stars by Zeus as the constellation Sagittarius (Centaurus). From there, as John Updike concluded in the epilogue to his 1964 allegorical novel The Centaur:

> he assists in the regulation of our destinies, though in this latter time few living mortals cast their eyes respectfully toward Heaven, and fewer still sit as students to the stars.[12]

References

1. Hyginus. *Fabulae (Fables) 100–149, Paragraph 138. The Myths of Hyginus.* Lawrence, KS, University of Kansas Press, 1960.
2. Hyginus. *Fabulae (Fables) Paragraph 274. The Myths of Hyginus.* Lawrence, KS, University of Kansas Press, 1960.
3. Pliny the Elder. *Natural History, The Loeb Classical Library.* Cambridge, MA, Harvard University Press, 1962.
4. Homer. *Iliad of Homer, 11.* Chicago, University of Chicago Press. Translated by: Lattimore R, 2011.
5. Panopolis No. *Dionysiaca, Loeb Classical Library.* Cambridge, MA, Harvard University Press, 1940.
6. Eliot Syr Thomas. *The Dictionary of Syr Thomas Eliot.* London, Thomas Bertheleti, 1538.
7. Machiavelli N. *The Prince; an Elizabethan Translation.* Chapel Hill, The University of North Carolina Press, 1944.
8. Hornblower S. *The Oxford Companion to Classical Civilization.* Oxford, Oxford University Press, 2004.
9. Zincgref JW. *Emblematum Ethico-Politicorum Centuria.* Heidelberg, Apud Clementem Ammonium, 1666.
10. Manilius. *Astronomica, Book 5 at 360. Loeb Classical Library.* Translated by Goold GP. Cambridge, MA, Harvard University Press, 1977, pp 328–31.
11. John of Salisbury Bishop of Chartres. *Policraticus: Frivolities of Courtiers and Footprints of Philosophers; Being a Translation of the First, Second, and Third Books and Selections from the Seventh and Eighth Books of John of Salisbury.* Translated by Pike, JB. New York, Octagon Books, 1972, p 436.
12. Updike J. *The Centaur. (Epilogue).* 1st Edition. New York, Knopf, 1963.

8
SKILL: *TEKHNE*

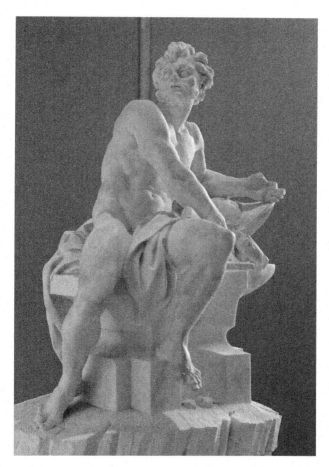

Vulcan. 1742. Guillaume Coustou the Younger (1716–1777). Seized during the French Revolution by Napoleon Bonaparte and exchanged in 1815. Reception piece for the French Royal Academy. (Guillaume Coustou the Younger, public domain, via Wikimedia Commons.)

Among the more mundane-sounding but consummately important requirements for the practice of anesthesiology is the ability to be procedurally deft – skillful, quick, and clever at the same time. Differences (and popularity!) between practitioners are readily apparent not only in their results, but also in their speed and facility, often called "smoothness," ability to engender confidence in their patients and colleagues, and availability of alternatives in case one method or approach is consistently unsuccessful. Anesthesiologists must be able to manage the airway in an expert fashion, support breathing with manual ventilation via a mask or a variety of other airway devices including endotracheal tubes. Their knowledge, familiarity and skill with a variety of instruments and pieces of equipment in order to accomplish this life-saving skill is crucial to the practice, as is the ability to access veins, arteries, and major vessels in the central circulation for special monitoring lines. A variety of other skills are critical as well, such as the ability to use ultrasound in the operating room or the intensive care unit, place a variety of nerve blocks to provide pain relief during obstetrical care or in the management of acute or chronic pain. The anesthetic care of infants and small children is a specific subspecialty within anesthesiology, demanding exquisitely dexterous skills in these areas. All of this is beyond the ongoing scholarship requirements for fund of knowledge and cognitive expertise, and is far from "mundane."

***

Tekhne was the spirit of art, technical skill and craft. She was closely associated with *Hephaistos* (*Vulcan*, L.) and the *Mousai* (the Muses). Unfortunately, artistic images of *Tekhne* do not exist. There is a literary reference to an altar to *Tekhne* in the ancient town of Gadeira (Gibraltar) in southern Spain.[1] *Tekhne* bridged the values personified by *Hephaistos* and the *Mousai* because her spirit embodied craft *and* art, emphasizing precision and skill; she was the personification of *precise* technique as an art form.

In a broad sense, *Tekhne* also extended beyond the visual arts to rhetoric and communication. Rhetoric, the art of persuasion, provided the rules and guidelines for writing effective speeches.

This skill was essential in a society where every Athenian citizen was expected to participate in the Assembly and be a persuasive public speaker if called upon. Would that every anesthesia practitioner had this requirement as a "technical" skill – the development of eloquence (see Chapter 20)!

Hephaistos

Hephaistos (Vulcan) was the god of fire and patron god of all artisans, blacksmiths, craftsmen, and sculptors. He was the manufacturer of art, arms, iron, jewelry and armor for various gods and heroes, including the thunderbolts of *Zeus*. He gave skill to mortal artists and was believed to have taught men the arts that embellish and adorn life. *Hephaistos* also created the first woman *Pandora*, whom he sculpted out of clay.

As skilled a craftsman as he was, he was also consistently described as ugly and deformed. Homer and Hesiod both characterized *Hephaistos* as "the cripple-foot god" and "the lame one." The cause of his malady was controversial; Homer described it as a congenital disorder, while an alternate description ascribed the lameness to injury after being forcibly ejected from the heavens by Zeus. This "ugliness" resulted in several amorous rejections.

The Muses

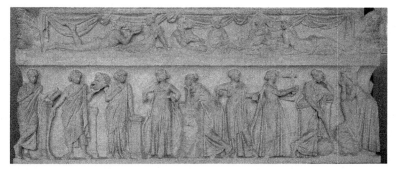

Sarcophagus known as the "Muses Sarcophagus," featuring the nine Muses and their attributes. From left to right: *Klio, Thalia, Erato, Euterpe, Polyhymnia, Kalliope, Terpsikhore, Urania* and *Melpomene*. (Louvre Museum, public domain, via Wikimedia Commons.)

The nine Mousai were each devoted to different aspects of the arts:

Klio	History
Thalia	Comedy
Erato	Love poetry
Euterpe	Music, Song, and Lyric Poetry
Polyhymnia	Hymns
Kalliope	Epic poetry
Terpsikhore	Dance
Urania	Astronomy
Melpomene	Tragedy

The role of the Muse was to *inspire* the art, not necessarily to *create* it. To "carry a mousa" is "to excel in the arts," according to the poet Pindar. Mousike (the root of "music") was just "one of the arts of the Muses." In the broad sense, the Muses inspired precise, pithy and articulate communication, historical perspective, a balance to the twists and turns of life (Comedy and Tragedy), and beauty in motion (Dance). The Histories of Herodotus (called the "Father of History" by Cicero) were divided into nine books, named after the nine Muses. For the poet Solon, the Muses brought prosperity and friendship; *he believed the Muses would help inspire people to do their best.* Ancient authors invoked the Muses when writing poetry, hymns or epic history. The invocation typically occurred near the beginning of their work, asking for help or inspiration, or simply inviting the Muse to sing directly *through* the author. For example, Homer, in Book I of *The Odyssey*, introduces the epic with:

> Sing to me of the man, Muse, the man of twists and turns
> driven time and again off course, once he had plundered
> the hallowed heights of Troy.[2]

and Virgil, in Book I of the *Aeneid*:

> O Muse! the causes and the crimes relate;
> What goddess was provok'd, and whence her hate;
> For what offense the Queen of Heav'n began
> To persecute so brave, so just a man.[3]

Other famous works by Ovid, Dante, Chaucer, Shakespeare and Milton included invocations of the Muse.

Homeric Hymn 20 invoked the creative spirit of the Muses to pay homage to the craft of *Hephaistos*:

> Sing, clear-voiced Muses, of Hephaistos famed for inventions. With bright-eyed Athene he taught men glorious gifts throughout the world – men who before used to dwell in caves in the mountains like wild beasts. But now that they have learned crafts through Hephaistos the famed worker, easily they live a peaceful life in their own houses the whole year round. Be gracious, Hephaistos, and grant me success and prosperity![4]

We could do worse than begin our medical endeavors with an invocation to a Muse, or hope that the creativity, artistry and precision of a Muse would flow through us to our work with patients!

***

Craft

Only relatively recently has the importance of craft seemed to lag behind intellect. This distinction blurs, not surprisingly, when one is in search of a particular skill or a skillful practitioner. It is perhaps no accident that craft has always struggled for its place; *Hephaistos* started out suffering the rejection of his mother *Hera* when he was literally cast away from Mt. Olympos at birth. That was the first time; it was repeated by *Zeus* after *Hephaistos*, notwithstanding the previous hurt, defended *Hera* against *Zeus* and suffered *Zeus*' rage. Even while suffering ongoing humiliation and insults at the hands of the other Olympian Gods and the faithlessness of his wife *Aphrodite*, *Hephaistos* was nevertheless sought after for his incomparable utensils, arms, and jewelry. Artisans always are.

Muses and Medicine

Physicians have long paralleled their interest in medicine with the arts. Among the more famous were the poet William Carlos Williams (also a general practitioner and pediatrician); playwright Anton Chekhov; satirist Francois Rabelais; political theorist John Locke; Arthur Conan Doyle, the creator of Sherlock Holmes; poets Percy Bysshe Shelley and John Keats, and novelists Gertrude Stein (who attended Johns Hopkins School of Medicine but dropped out in her fourth year), William Somerset Maugham (who completed medical school at St. Thomas' Hospital), and James Joyce (who attended medical school in France but quickly dropped out).

Many non-famous physicians feel a strong, creative "link" to the arts that inspires their practice. Why?

Craft and Knowledge

Tekhne was paired with *Epistêmê*, or Knowledge. This exaggerated separation of practice and knowledge is useful because it identifies a dialectic as care becomes more centrifugally distributed to assistants, extenders and other para-medical practitioners.

This separation is poignantly underscored by the terms postgraduate medical *education* and residency *training*. There are those who argue that within the training/practice domain, skill acquisition is the principal need, relegating formal education to the lecture hall or classroom, where patient care is not directly provided. Aristotle outlined the basis for our modern contrast between epistêmê as pure theory and technê as practice. Yet even Aristotle referred to technê or craft as itself also epistêmê or knowledge because it is a practice grounded in an "account" – something involving theoretical understanding. There is an innate positive relationship between epistêmê and technê, as well as a fundamental contrast – a dialectic.

"Clinical teaching," especially that which occurs in dynamic real-time environments like the operating room, has been the subject of recent publications related to surgery, anesthesiology, interventional radiology, cardiology and emergency medicine. Such dynamic environments have to strike a balance between cognitive teaching and practical, often urgent, procedurally based interventions, where taking the time to step back and "teach" might be considered clinically dangerous for patient care. This is a difficult balance to achieve. The crucible of medical practice, however, involves the systematic and smooth integration of a cognitive fund of knowledge at the service of craft. Intriguingly, there is exquisite congruence as well as basic contrast between the two. By explicating this conundrum, Hephaistos as a personification integrates and validates their simultaneity, indeed, their necessity, in practice.

The incorporation of knowledge-based questions during clinical instruction is often caustically referred to as "pimping" – a form of questioning of junior colleagues by a person in power that affirms a hierarchal order in medicine (or in any training relationship).[5] But pimping is not the same as Socratic instruction, when questions and follow-up questions lead the learner to solve the problem him or her-self. While pimping uses the power of status to embarrass and humiliate the learner in a group environment, Socratic questions have as their goal the stepwise formation of critical thinking. However, Socratic teaching is time-consuming. Nevertheless, the fluid navigation between craft and knowledge, between Teknne and Epistêmê, the balance between the precision art of Hephaistos and Teknne and the scholarship of Kheiron and the inspiration of the Muses, is the ideal of the skilled clinician.

More importantly, the combination of knowledge and skill in the clinical setting is crucial because often, the physical action "fixes" the knowledge base better than either one alone.[6]

References

1. Philostratus the Athenian. *The Life of Apollonius of Tyana, the Epistles of Apollonius and the Treatise of Eusebius, Loeb Classical Library*. New York, The Macmillan Co, 1912.
2. Homer. *The Odyssey*. New York, Viking, 1996, l. 541.
3. Virgil. *Aeneid*. London, Folio Society, 1993, l. 417.
4. Hesiod. *Homeric Hymns and Homerica, The Loeb Classical Library*. Cambridge, MA, Harvard University Press, 1914, l. 657.
5. Oh R, Reamy B. The Socratic method and pimping: optimizing the use of stress and fear in instruction. *AMA Journal of Ethics* 2014; 16: 182–186.
6. Busan A. Learning styles of medical students – implications in education. *Current Health Sciences Journal* 2014; 40: 104–110.

9
BEAUTY AND GRACE: *KALLEIS*, *APHRODITE* AND *APOLLO*

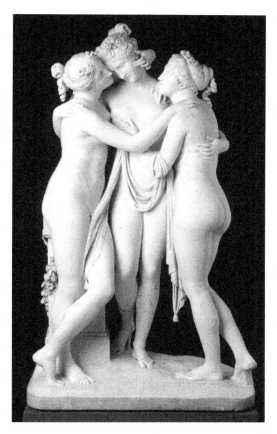

From youngest to oldest, the *Kharites* (*Gratiae*, or Graces, Roman) were: *Agleaea*, also known as *Kalleis* ("Beauty"), *Euphrosyne* ("Good Cheer") and *Thalia* ("Festivities"). *Kalleis* is in the center. Antonio Canova (1757–1822). The Three Graces (1813–1816). (Hermitage Museum.)

DOI: 10.1201/9781003201328-12

It is surprising that grace and beauty are infrequently incorporated into descriptions of medical care, especially for the procedurally-based specialties. I have vivid memories of my surgery and anesthesiology mentors instructing me on the proper way to hold my hands, tie knots, cut sutures, how to angle my wrist and countless other seemingly miniscule ergonomic corrections so that I could optimally – and effectively – position myself for success with a minimum of effort and time. Moreover, the all-too-frequent loss of grace in contemporary interactions with patients and colleagues is not only tragic but is also a common source of bad feelings easily leading to patient complaint, peer disputes and legal actions. For the Ancients, values associated with beauty and grace were *integral* to the professions as well as all social interactions. These values were incorporated into daily life, personified as *Kalleis* (*Aglaea*), *Aphrodite* (*Venus*) and *Apollon* (*Apollo*).

Kalleis

Kalleis (*Aglaea*), in ancient Greek religion, was one of the *Kharites* (Graces, Roman), daughters of *Zeus* (*Jupiter*) and *Eurynome*. *Kalleis*, also known as *Kharis* and *Aglaea*, the youngest of the three *Kharites*, was the goddess of beauty, splendor, glory and adornment. *Kalleis* was married to *Hephaistos* after his divorce from *Aphrodite*[1] and she was the mother of four younger *Kharites*. Her older sisters were *Euphrosyne*, the goddess of joy or mirth, and *Thalia*, the goddess of festivity and lavish banquets.[2] The sisters were attendants to *Aphrodite*, the goddess of love, with *Kalleis* sometimes acting as her messenger. Individually, the *Kharites* represented qualities that were both honored and awed by the Greeks, charm and grace.

Pindar, in Olympian Ode 14.1 suggested the importance of incorporating beauty into worklife[3]:

> Whose haunts are by Kephissos' (Cephisus') river, you queens (the Kharites) beloved of poets' song, ruling Orkhomenos (Orchomenus),* that sunlit city and land of lovely steeds,

---

* A river with its headwaters on the northern slopes of Mount Parnassos (Parnassus) and the southern foothills of the Mount Othrys, emptying into Lake Kopais (Copais) near the town of Orkhomenos (Orchomenus) in Boeotia (central Greece).

watch and ward of the ancient Minyan race, hear now my prayer, you Kharites (Charites, Graces) three.

For in your gift are all our mortal joys, and every sweet thing, be it wisdom, beauty, or glory, that *makes rich the soul of man.* Nor even can the immortal gods order at their behest the dance and festals,[†] lacking the Kharites' aid; who are the steward of all rites of heaven, whose thrones are set at Pytho[‡] beside Apollon of the golden bow, and who with everlasting honour worship the Father, lord of great Olympos.

Euphrosyne, lover of song, and Aglaia (Aglaea) revered, daughters of Zeus the all-highest, hearken, and with Thalia, darling of harmony, look on our songs of revel, on light feet stepping to grace this happy hour ...

Was this a *forme fruste* of understanding burnout – the loss of joy and engagement, in effect, the loss of the component of "richness" and beauty in daily work? Richness is achieved – or perceived – in the presence of beauty and grace, more so than the possession of mere knowledge or technical skill.

Aphrodite

Aphrodite (Venus, Roman) was the goddess of love, beauty, desire, and pleasure. Although married to Hephaistos she had many lovers, notably *Ares (Mars)*, *Adonis,* and *Anchises.* Her beauty was beyond description and she, of all the goddesses, was most likely to appear nude or seminude. Poets praised the radiance of her smile and her laughter. Her symbols included roses and other flowers, the scallop shell, and the myrtle wreath.

In keeping with the Greek dialectic, Attic (classical) philosophers of the 4th century BCE separated a "celestial" Aphrodite (*Aprodite Urania*) of transcendent principles with the "common" Aphrodite of the people (*Aphrodite Pandemos*).[4] *Aphrodite Urania* represented the love of body and soul, while *Aphrodite Pandemos* was associated only with carnal love. In effect, Aphrodite was two goddesses, one older the other younger.[5] This dual personification provides a context for understanding the *maturation of love with time. Aphrodite's* dual

---

† Medieval form of feast or festival.
‡ Ancient name for Delphi.

nature was revealed when she immaturely punished those who neglected her worship or despised her power, while at the same time she favored and protected others to repay their homage to her.

Aphrodite was married to *Hephaistos*, who married *Kharis* following *Aphrodite*'s infidelity in her affair with *Ares*. Despite her self-indulgence and infidelity, above all, Aphrodite was the goddess of love and beauty. Her paradoxical nature – wives and courtesans each established cults for her – may be the reason why ancient authors distinguished between several *Aphrodites*.

In accordance with the Ancient poets, *Aphrodite* had no childhood. In every portrayal and in each reference, she is born as an adult, nubile and infinitely desirable. In many of the late anecdotal myths, she was characterized as vain, ill-tempered and easily offended. In stark contrast to her husband, *Hephaistos*, one of the most even-tempered of the deities, she was frequently unfaithful. As Homer related in the Odyssey, *Aphrodite* seemed to prefer *Ares*, the volatile god of war, as she was attracted to his violent nature.

Apollon

Apollon (Apollo) was the god of light, music, arts, knowledge, healing, plague and darkness, prophecy, poetry, purity, athleticism, manly beauty, and enlightenment. He was the son of *Zeus* and *Leto* and the twin brother of *Artemis* (*Diana*, Roman), the chaste huntress. *Apollo* and *Artemis* were identified with the sun and moon (respectively); both used a bow and arrow. In sculpture, *Apollo* was depicted as the ideal of the *kouros* (a beardless, athletic youth), with long hair and an ideal physique.

The most beautiful and celebrated among the existing representations of *Apollo* is the Apollo of Belvedere. The god is represented with commanding yet serene majesty; the forehead is higher than in other ancient figures, suggesting intellect and on it there is a pair of locks, while the rest of his hair flows freely down on his neck, portraying confident physical beauty. His figure is lithe rather than overbearing. While he was accorded laudatory epithets:

> The god who affords help and wards off evil.
> The god of prophecy.
> The god of song and music.

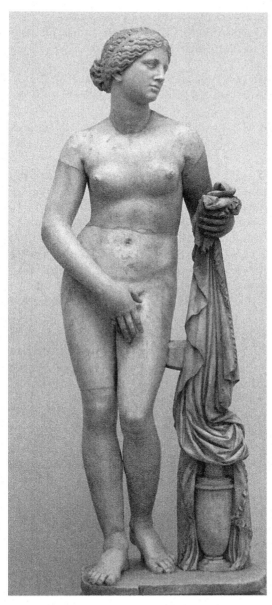

Cnidus Aphrodite. Copy of Praxiteles, 4th century. (Museo nazionale romano di palazzo Altemps, public domain, via Wikimedia Commons.)

The god who protects the flocks and cattle.
The god who delights in the foundation of towns and the establishment of civil constitutions.

he could also be cruel and destructive, in true dialectical form and in contrast with his associated adulations:

the god who punishes and destroys ("*oulios*" – deadly) the wicked and overbearing.

This was in stark contrast to the family of Asklepios whose members were solely devoted to healing (see Chapter 2). *Apollo* could punish – brutally – as well as heal and purify. He slew the Giant *Tityus* for trying to rape *Leto*, his mother, and massacred *Niobe*'s children because they insulted *Leto*. He didn't tolerate the appearance of betrayal; this he had in common with *Aphrodite*. With great power not only came great responsibility – but also great aggression. Although always held as an ideal, especially for rational thought, and often contrasted with the emotional lability of *Dionysus*, *Apollo* was also vengeful.

Apollo shot arrows infected with the plague into the Greek encampment during the Trojan War in retribution for Agamemnon's insult to Khryses, a priest of *Apollo*, whose daughter Khryseis had been captured, providing the first mythological accounting of biological weapons.

When *Zeus* struck down *Apollo*'s son *Asklepios* with a lightning bolt for resurrecting *Hippolytus* from the dead, *Apollo* in revenge killed the *Cyclopes*, *Hephaistos*' smiths, who had fashioned the lightning bolt for *Zeus*. *Apollo* would have been banished forever for this but was instead sentenced to one year of hard labor due to the intercession of his mother, *Leto*.

Apollo had menacing traits aside from his plague-bringing, death-dealing arrows. *Marsyas* was a satyr[§] who challenged *Apollo* to a contest of music. He had found an *aulos* (double oboe) on the ground, tossed away after its invention by *Athena* because it made her cheeks puffy. The contest was judged by the *Muses*. After they each performed, both were deemed equal until *Apollo*

[§] One of a class of lustful, drunken woodland gods. In Greek art they were represented as a man with a horse's ears and tail.

BEAUTY AND GRACE 97

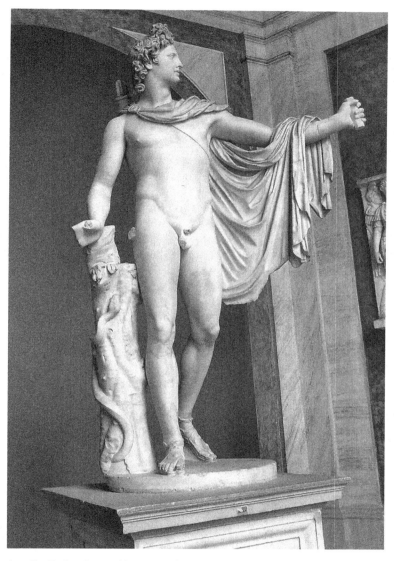

Apollo Belvedere. The youthful god Apollo stands nude beside a serpent-entwined pillar with his arm outstretched. Marble. Roman copy of Greek bronze statue by Leochares 350–325 BC. (After Leochares, public domain, via Wikimedia Commons.)

decreed they play and sing at the same time. Because *Apollo* played the lyre, this was easy to do. *Marsyas* could not do this, as he only knew how to use the flute and could not sing at the same time. *Apollo* was declared the winner because of this. *Apollo* flayed *Marsyas* alive for his hubris in challenging a god.

He often appeared in the company of the *Muses*, illustrating his intimate association with their artistic inspiration. As their leader (*Apollon Musegetes*) and director of their choir, *Apollo* functioned as the patron god of music and poetry. *Hermes* created the lyre for him, and the instrument became a common attribute of *Apollo*. In the Iliad he entertained the gods by playing the phorminx, the earliest form of lyre, during their feast. The association of the lyre with the poet is that the two complement each other as forms of communication. This association with beautiful, alternate forms of communication, poetry and music, underscores the importance of diversity of communication as a characteristic of the god of healing.

As the patron of Delphi (*Pythian Apollo*), *Apollo* was an oracular god – the prophetic deity of the Delphic Oracle.** This was in keeping with the value held highest by *Hippocrates* in medical practice – prognostication. In Classical Greece, *Apollo* was the god of light and of music, but in popular religion he also functioned to keep away evil, which suggested an important role for health maintenance and the promotion of what we would now recognize as wellness

Apollo as healer was connected with *Paean*, the physician of the Gods in the Iliad. He was the personification of the holy magic-song sung by the magician-physicians. This invocation was supposed to cure disease, and later became a noun for a hymn or song, "paean." *Apollo* was said to have sent a plague to the Achaeans. To appease *Apollo*, and in search of a cure, the Achaeans prayed with a song and called their own god, the *Paean*. About the 4th century BCE, the paean became a song of adulation; its object was either to implore protection against disease and misfortune or to offer thanks after such protection had been rendered. It became the Roman custom, for example, for a paean to be sung by an army on the march and before entering

---

** A person through whom a deity is believed to speak the prophecies of the Delphic *oracle*, or an authoritative or wise expression or answer.

into battle, when a fleet left the harbor, and also after a victory had been won.

***

Apollo represented the beauty and grace of harmony, order, and reason – characteristics contrasted with those of Dionysus, god of wine, who represented ecstasy and disorder. This dialectic persists as the adjectives Apollonian (the rational, ordered and self-disciplined aspects of human nature) and Dionysian (the sensual, spontaneous, and emotional aspects of human nature). In the arts, a distinction is sometimes made between the Apollonian and Dionysian impulses where the former is concerned with imposing intellectual order and the latter with chaotic creativity. Friedrich Nietzsche argued that a fusion of the two was most desirable. The Greeks also thought of the two qualities as complementary because the two gods were brothers.

Albert Szent-Györgyi, a Hungarian biochemist who won the Nobel Prize in Physiology or Medicine in 1937, recognized that "a discovery must be, by definition, at variance with existing knowledge," and divided scientists into two categories – the Apollonians and the Dionysians. He called scientific dissenters, who explored the fringes of knowledge Dionysians, writing

> in science the Apollonian tends to develop established lines to perfection, while the Dionysian rather relies on intuition and is more likely to open new, unexpected alleys for research ... The future of mankind depends on the progress of science, and the progress of science depends on the support it can find. Support mostly takes the form of grants, and the present methods of distributing grants unduly favor the Apollonian.[6]

References

1. Hesiod. *The Homeric Hymns and Homerica. Theogony.* In. Evelyn-White H, trans. Cambridge, MA, Harvard University Press, 1914, Lines 945 ff.
2. Hesiod. *The Homeric Hymns and Homerica. Theogony.* Cambridge, MA, Harvard University Press, 1914.
3. Pindar. *Odes of Pindar: Olympian Ode 14.* In. Conway G, Stoneman R, trans. London, J.M. Dent, 1997, p 434.
4. Plato. Symposium. In. *Oxford Approaches to Classical Literature.* Oxford, Oxford University Press Hunter, RL, 2004, 181a–d.

5. Hunter R. *Plato's Symposium*. New York, Oxford University Press, 2004, p 44.
6. Szent-Gyorgi A. Dionysians and Apollonians: letter from Albert Szent-Gyorgi to Science. Science. 1972; 176(4038): 966.

10
WISDOM: *SOPHIA*

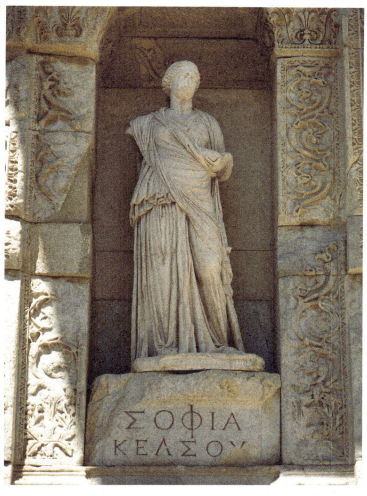

Sophia, personification of wisdom at the Library of Celsus in Ephesus (second century).

Originally associated with cleverness or skill (the literal translation of *sophos*), a valued trait among the gods, *Sophia* later came to represent wisdom and intelligence in parallel with the development of Platonic "philosophy" ("love of Sophia," or wisdom). A dialectic is once again evident by making distinctions between *sophia* (skill with regard to handicraft and art) and *phronesis* (sound judgment, intelligence and practical action). Phronesis was subtly different than two other concepts introduced earlier in Chapter 8 – tekhne and epistēmē – providing a bridge that might be called *pragmatism*. Others have claimed an equivalency for the more currently fashionable term *mindfulness*.[1]

The incorporation of *virtue* provided an additional dimension to wisdom, illustrated by the Section 2 figure of *Arete*. *Sophia* was a combination of the Classical notion of *nous*, intellect with the ability to understand and discern reality, and *epistēmē*, teachable knowledge, sometimes equated with science. In other contexts, *nous* has been equated with common sense and awareness, all integral to successful clinical medicine.

In medicine, wisdom and intelligence augment mere knowledge by allowing it to be molded to the needs of an individual within a specific context. This is the essence of clinical wisdom and judgement and it gives depth to mere knowledge.[2,3]

***

Knowledge deities were also associated with wisdom and intelligence in addition to knowledge. In Greek mythology, the knowledge deities included:

- *Apollo*, Olympian god of light, music, poetry, knowledge and the sun.
- the *Muses*, personifications of knowledge, wisdom and the arts
- *Athena*, Olympian goddess of wisdom, architecture, art, war strategy, and civilization
- *Koios*, Titan of intellect
- *Hephaestus*, Olympian god of invention and fire
- *Metis*, Oceanid of wisdom and wise counsel
- *Prometheus*, Titan of forethought
- *Phoebe*, Titan of prophecy

- *Hekate*, Goddess of sorcery, magic, witchcraft, necromancy, ghosts, prophecy, fire, light, crossroads, darkness, night, the moon, wilderness, and dogs

Knowledge deities represented a broad range of key concepts, which added texture and dimension to knowledge, illustrated by the many epithets attached to their names. Knowledge concerned itself not only with facts and information but also the *capacity to acquire such facts* (intellect) and the judgment to apply such knowledge wisely.

Intellect

Koios (*"query, questioning"*)

Koios was also one of the Titans, the giant sons and daughters of *Ouranos* (Uranus; Heaven) and *Gaia* (Earth). Like most of the Titans, he was also important for his descendants. *Koios* fathered *Leto* and *Asteria* with his sister *Phoebe*, associated with the translation "shining" (*phoebus*). Given that "shining" *Phoebe* symbolized prophetic wisdom just as *Koios* represented rational intelligence, the couple may have functioned together as avatars for knowledge and wisdom. Along with the other Titans, *Koios* was overthrown by *Zeus* and the other Olympians in the *Titanomachy** ("Titan Battle"). Afterwards, he and all his brothers were imprisoned in Tartarus by *Zeus*. *Koios*, later overcome with madness, broke free from his bonds and attempted to escape his imprisonment, but was repelled by *Cerberus*.[4] Thus, power overwhelmed authority.

As a Titan of wisdom and prophecy, *Koios* was also a god of heavenly oracles. He was believed to be hearing prophetic voices of his father *Ouranos* (heaven), just like *Phoebe* heard prophetic voices of her mother *Gaia* (earth). Together they had two daughters who inherited the powers of their parents. *Leto* was a goddess of modesty and motherhood and was associated with *prophetic power of light and heaven*, while *Asteria* was associated with *prophetic power of night and the dead*. This prophecy dialectic was

---

* A ten-year series of battles fought in Thessaly between the Titans fighting against the Olympians to decide which generation of gods would reign over the Universe; it ended in victory for the Olympians.

also passed to their descendants. *Apollo* inherited the power of the light from his mother *Leto*, while *Hekate* inherited the power of the night from *Asteria*. Perhaps, this is why *Koios* was identified as the Titan of intellect. Having knowledge is one thing, but the ability to understand and apply such knowledge toward predicting the future – prognostication – is wisdom according to a central aphorism of *Hippocratic* medicine:

> For by foreseeing and foretelling, in the presence of the sick, the present, the past, and the future, and explaining the omissions which patients have been guilty of, he will be the more readily believed to be acquainted with the circumstances of the sick; so that men will have confidence to entrust themselves to such a physician ... He will manage the cure best who has foreseen what is to happen from the present state of matters.[5]

Knowledge

The roles of *Apollo* and the *Muses* were examined earlier in Chapters 2 and 9 in conjunction with the family of *Asklepios* as well as Beauty and Grace.

Wisdom

Athena (Minerva; Roman)

Athena was the wise companion of heroes and the patron goddess of heroic actions. As *Athena Promachos* ("Athena who fights in the front line") she was first in battle.[6] Literally, she represented command, leadership and courage. Figuratively, she was the disciplined, strategic side of war, in contrast to her brother *Ares*, the patron of violence, slaughter and maiming – the "raw forces of war."[7] Although a goddess of war strategy and a leader of troops, *she preferred the use of wisdom to settle conflicts.*

Homer referred to Athena epithetically as *Glaukopis*, ("bright-eyed" or "with gleaming eyes"); glaúx ("little owl") has the same etymology. Athena is frequently depicted with an owl perched on her hand. Even today the owl is a symbol of wisdom.[8] A more poetic usage of "bright-eyed" could easily refer to clairvoyance, vision, or prophesy.

In the context of contemporary medical practice, particularly anesthesiology practice, one can easily invoke wisdom, experience, judgment and prognostication daily when balancing the asynchronous role of being in-the-moment in the operating room as well as forecasting ("prognosticating") what is likely to happen in the next few minutes if the bleeding continues, the blood pressure decreases, the blood saturation starts to decrease, etc. Clinical practice in the operating room is a constant shift of asynchronous prognostications between the present and the future.

Metis

Metis ("wisdom," "skill," or "craft") was an Oceanid,[†] from the generation of Titans before the gods of Olympos and was the first spouse of *Zeus*. As an epithet, a form of her name (*Mêtieta*; "the wise counselor") was attached to *Zeus* in the Homeric poems, although *metis* included both wisdom and cunning, an intriguing combination highly regarded by Athenians. This fusion was both a threat to *Zeus* as well as an indispensable aid:

> Now Zeus, king of the gods, made Metis his wife first, and *she was wisest* among gods and mortal men. But when she was about to bring forth the goddess bright-eyed Athena, Zeus craftily deceived her with cunning words and put her in his own belly, as Earth and starry Heaven advised. For they advised him so, to the end that *no other should hold royal sway over the eternal gods in place of Zeus*; for very wise children were destined to be born of her, first the maiden bright-eyed Tritogeneia,[‡] equal to her father in strength and in wise understanding; but afterwards she was to bear a son of overbearing spirit, king of gods and men. But Zeus put her into his own belly first, that the goddess might devise for him both good and evil.[9]

[†] Sea nymphs who were the three thousand daughters of the Titans Oceanus and Tethys.

[‡] An epithet in association with Athena, related to Athena's birth from the head of Zeus, thereby inheriting his wise understanding.

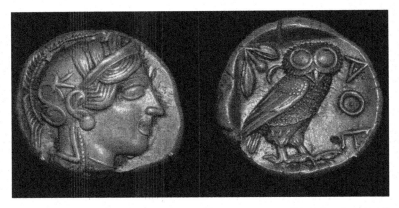

Athenian 'owl' tetradrachm, late 5th century BC. An Athenian 'owl' tetradrachm with the head of Athena on one side, and her owl on the other, late 5th century BC.

Zeus must have been pretty desperate to silence Metis, yet he was too late and her influence would not be stilled.

Prophecy

Prometheus

The Titan *Prometheus* ("forethought") was known as the greatest benefactor of humanity. The legendary compassionate stories of the creation of man from clay as well as the diversion of culinary delicacies from the Olympian gods to humanity were eclipsed by his theft of fire from Olympos for the benefit of mankind. The enraged *Zeus* punished *Prometheus* by chaining him to a rock for eternity, where his liver was eaten daily by an eagle, only to be regenerated at night due to his immortality.

The Prometheus myth was first described in Hesiod's Theogony:

> Now Iapetus took to wife the neat-ankled maid Clymene, daughter of Ocean, and went up with her into one bed. And she bore him a stout-hearted son, Atlas: also she bore very glorious Menoetius and *clever Prometheus, full of various wiles*, and scatter-brained Epimetheus who from the first was a mischief to men who eat bread; for it was he who first took

WISDOM: *SOPHIA* 107

of Zeus the woman, the maiden whom he had formed...
And ready-witted *Prometheus he bound with inextricable bonds, cruel chains, and drove a shaft through his middle, and set on him a long-winged eagle, which used to eat his immortal liver; but by night the liver grew as much again everyway as the long-winged bird devoured in the whole day...because Prometheus matched himself in wit with the almighty son of Cronos.*[10]

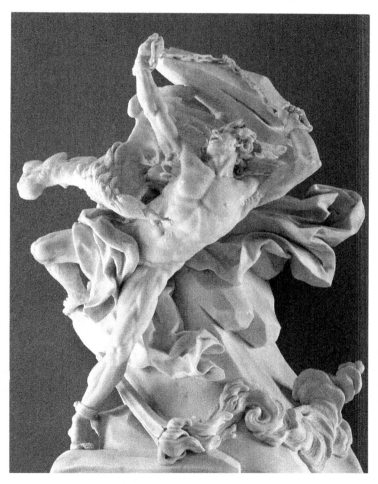

Prometheus depicted in a sculpture by Nicolas-Sébastien Adam, 1762. (Louvre, Public domain, via Wikimedia Commons.)

His name signified "forethought," in contrast to his brother *Epimetheus* (the husband of Pandora), whose name meant "afterthought." In the Theogony, Hesiod portrays *Prometheus* as a challenger to *Zeus's* omnipotence. To understand the role of *Prometheus* in his struggle with *Zeus* is to understand the struggle between generations, symbolic of parents eventually giving ground to the growing needs, vitality, and responsibilities of the new generation in order to perpetuate society. This aspect of (social) forethought is amplified by knowledge-based forethought – prognostication.

Prometheus re-emerged as a literature avatar after the Renaissance and the advance of science. Mary Shelley's science-fiction horror story "Frankenstein" (published in 1818) was subtitled "The Modern Prometheus" – a literary reminder of the time context. The influence of the myth of *Prometheus* extends well into the 20th and 21st century and hovers as an allegorical reminder of the perilous cost of how knowledge and forethought can challenge established authority with resulting dire consequences. Far less threatening to be Epimetheus than Prometheus.

Phoebe and Hekate

Phoebe ("shining") was also one of the original Titans. Given the meaning of her name and her association with the Delphic oracle, *Phoebe* could easily be viewed as the Titan goddess of prophecy and oracular intellect. Through *Leto*, her daughter, she was the grandmother of *Apollo* and *Artemis*, and through her other daughter *Asteria*, the grandmother of *Hekate*. *Phoebe* and *Hekate* represented the dialectic of prophecy, good and bad, fortunate and unfortunate.

Hekate was the goddess of crossroads, entryways, light, magic, witchcraft, knowledge of herbs and poison plants, necromancy[§] and sorcery. These epithets easily lend themselves to dual interpretations of *Hekate's* role – good and bad prophecy, or fortune

---

[§] Communicating with the dead, especially in order to predict the future.

and misfortune. As a Chthonic** goddess, *Hekate* was held in high regard by Hesiod although her reputation was spotty amongst other writers. Shrines to Hekate were placed at doorways to homes as well as cities with the belief that she would protect from restless dead and other spirits. Likewise, shrines to *Hekate* were placed at three way crossroads.

***

According to Hippocrates' Prognostic 1:

> It seems to be highly desirable that a physician should pay much attention to prognosis. If he is able to tell his patients when he visits them not only about their past and present symptoms, but also to tell them what is going to happen, as well as to fill in the details they have omitted, he will increase his reputation as a medical practitioner and people will have no qualms in putting themselves under his care. Moreover, he will be better be able to effect a cure if he can foretell, from the present symptoms, the future course of the disease.[11]

Exquisitely practiced in anesthesiology but common to all medical practice is the duality of synchronous and asynchronous attention, which involves living in the present but also forecasting into the future. In anesthesiology the stakes are high and immediate – a failure to be mindful and attentive in real-time may lead to mortal consequences right before your eyes, while a failure to be future-oriented may misinform an anticipated strategy or intervention that would magnify a problem 10 minutes hence. Timelines in many specialties are longer than that, but the short-interval horizons in the operating room are appealing to some and frightening to many. As soon as a patient is seen preoperatively, the anesthetist has to think of customizing an induction

---

** Chthonic ("in, under, or beneath the earth") literally means "subterranean," but the word in English describes deities or spirits of the underworld. The Greek word *khthon* is one of several for "earth"; it typically refers to that which is under the earth rather than the living surface of the land.

sequence in accordance with the patient's history and demands of the procedure. As soon as the induction of anesthesia begins, one has to look assiduously for potential adverse effects, and as soon as the likely period for those side effects passes thoughts are devoted simultaneously to intraoperative assessment as well as planning for the end of the anesthetic and optimal outcomes for the postoperative period. This demands wisdom in all of its broad definitions and also meets the Hippocratic value of prognostication as the highest fiduciary duty of medical practice.

Such prognostications come from intelligence, knowledge, and wisdom.

References

1. McEvilley T. *The Shape of Ancient Thought: Comparative Studies in Greek and Indian Philosophies.* New York, Allworth Press, 2002.
2. Kienle G, Kiene H. Clinical judgement and the medical profession. *Journal of Evaluation in Clinical Practice.* 2011; 17: 621–27.
3. Tversky A, Kahneman D. Judgment under uncertainty: Heuristics and biases. *Science* 1974; 185: 1124–31.
4. Flaccus V. Argonautica. In. Mozley J, trans. *Loeb Classical Library.* Vol 286. Cambridge, MA, Harvard University Press, 1928.
5. Hippocrates. Hippocratic Writings. In: Lloyd G, ed. Chadwick J, Mann W, Lonie I, Withington E, trans. London, Penguin Classics, 1983, 170.
6. Darmon J. *The Powers of War: Athena and Ares in Greek Mythology.* Chicago, IL, University of Chicago Press, 1992.
7. Herrington C. *Athena Parthenos and Athena Polias.* Manchester, Manchester University Press, 1955.
8. Deacy S, Villing A. *Athena in the Classical World.* Leiden, The Netherlands, Koninklijke Brill NV, 2001.
9. Hesiod. Theogony. in: Evelyn-White H, trans. London, William Heinemann Ltd, 1914, lines 885–99.
10. Hesiod. Theogony. in: *Evelyn-White H, trans.* London, William Heinemann Ltd, 1914, lines 507–44.
11. Lloyd G. *Hippocratic Writings.* New York, Penguin Books, 1983.

Part III

THE EMOTIONS

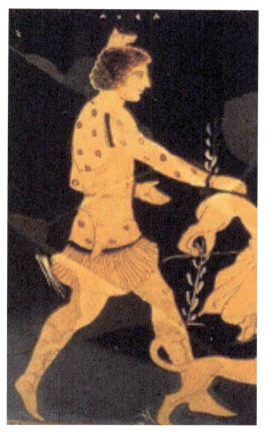

Lyssa was the goddess or personified spirit (*daimona*) of mad rage, fury and crazed frenzy. Note the dog headcap – representing the madness of rabies. *Lyssa* was closely related to the *Maniai* (*Maniae*), the goddesses of mania and madness. (Detail from an Athenian red-figure krater C5th BCE, Museum of Fine Arts Boston.) (www.mfa.org/)

DOI: 10.1201/9781003201328-14

There was no Greek overarching god, goddess or spirit for "emotions" because each of the deities was associated with their own emotional complexions and complexities. Daemones (personified spirits) of the human condition often represented emotions as abstract concepts, in addition to attributing specific emotions to particular gods.

Yet "emotional," often used in a pejorative sense when applied to difficulties in human interaction, can be devastating in any work setting. The operating room is no exception and in many ways is a most challenging crucible for navigating emergency situations if conflict and anger arise. The mastery of those feelings in the service of effective medical care constitutes an important aspect and challenge of professionalism.

11
STRIFE AND HARMONY: *ERIS* AND *HARMONIA*

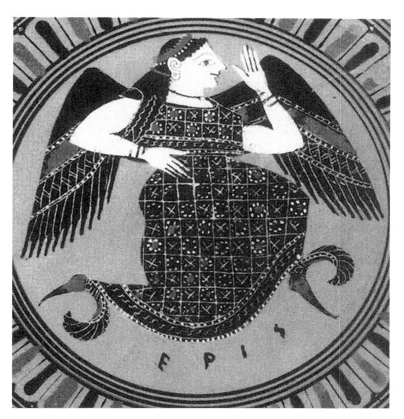

Eris on an Attic plate, ca. 575–525 BC.

DOI: 10.1201/9781003201328-15

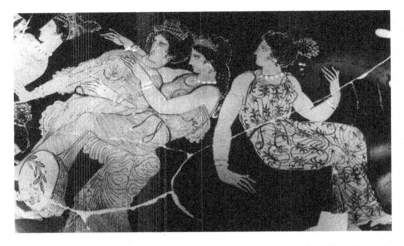

Three of the younger *Kharites* (Graces) – *Eudaimonia* (Happiness), *Harmonia* (Harmony) and *Paidia* (Play) – they were members of the retinue of Aphrodite. (From the National Archaeological Museum of Florence, attributed to Meidias Painter, ca. 450–400 BC.)

***

Harmony and Strife are constant accompaniments to modern medical care, particularly in the operating room, the crucible of interprofessional collaboration. "Spirited" debates often turn to internecine intellectual warfare as independence of thought and action – turf – is defended. While surgeons are often identified as the major source of "disruptive behavior,"[1] it is hardly their exclusive province. Sometimes the resolution of the debate is accomplished under guise of the "captain of the ship" doctrine, when the surgeon is "in charge" and exercises both authority and power. Other approaches may include collaboration, discussion and negotiation. Sometimes all parties declare victory and retreat, and occasionally revenge is delayed until another day. Regardless of the strategies and tactics for resolution, conflict itself impairs clarity of thought and judgment and undermines attention to patient care during critical periods. Shifting the focus from the patient to the surgeon or any individual or subgroup increases errors, may deter staff and medical trainees from pursuing careers in the operating room, frequently decreases respect for surgeons, engenders bad feelings (powerlessness, worthlessness and frustration), and interrupts attention and learning. This is the subject of much conflict resolution training going on in medical education and amongst medical staffs.[2,3]

When viewed from "systems theory" rather than strictly interpersonally, conflict often results from the composition and (dys)function of operating room teams, equipment management, and (dis)engagement of the administrative leadership of the operating room. "Stable" teams are well recognized as facilitating surgical results because of established working patterns, familiarity with procedures and equipment and patterned styles of communication, but are also challenging because they require significant customizing of available schedules, are surgeon-centric, and expose the operating room staff to uneven levels of experience when all must take emergency call with other specialties. Such teams may also, because of unwitting and unintentional collusion, "cover" for their surgeons' lack of professional behaviors when interacting with other teams or administrative leadership. In contrast, leaders (surgeons, or not) who demonstrate effective management of the emotional milieu of a volatile situation increase trust and enhance team performance.[4] Simulation has added a new dimension to this because of the chance to stop, debrief, step outside of traditionally stratified roles, and "practice" conflict resolution.

Conflict may have positive aspects as well; not all conflict is destructive.[5] Indeed, in specific circumstances, often resembling the group effort in the operating room (a high-functioning group performing a nonroutine task), disagreements about the tasks have fewer detrimental effects. In some cases, such disagreements are actually beneficial.[6] While strife cannot necessarily be counted on as a sustainable form of "energizing" conflict resolution, there is something to be said for Lincoln's successful "Team of Rivals" approach.[7] His success was largely attributable to "empathetic intelligence" – in addition to his position of power as President.

***

Eris (Strife)

Harmonia is the immortal goddess of harmony. Her Roman counterpart is *Concordia*, and her Greek opposite is *Eris*, whose Roman counterpart is *Discordia*.

In Hesiod's *Works and Days*,[8] *two* different goddesses named Eris were recognized:

> So, after all, there was not one kind of Strife alone, but all over the earth there are two. As for the one, a man would praise her when he came to understand her; but the other is blameworthy: and they are wholly different in nature. For one fosters evil war and battle, being cruel: *her no man loves*; but perforce, through the will of the deathless gods, *men pay harsh Strife her honour due*. But the other is the elder daughter of dark Night (Nyx), and the son of Cronus who sits above and dwells in the aether, set her in the roots of the earth: and she is far kinder to men. *She stirs up even the shiftless to toil*; for a man grows eager to work when he considers his neighbour, a rich man who hastens to plough and plant and put his house in good order; and neighbour vies with his neighbour as he hurries after wealth. This Strife is wholesome for men. And potter is angry with potter, and craftsman with craftsman, and beggar is jealous of beggar, and minstrel of minstrel.

This nuanced personification is the dialectic of Strife, not an antilogy to Harmony but a reflection of the energy derived from challenge and struggle, fueling ambition and competition.

In Hesiod's *Theogony*,[9] Strife, the daughter of Night, is less kindly spoken of as she brings forth other traits in her personified children:

> But abhorred *Eris* ("Strife") bare painful *Ponos* ("Toil/Labor"), *Lethe* ("Forgetfulness") and *Limos* ("Famine") and tearful *Algea* ("Pains/Sorrows"), *Hysminai* ("Fightings/Combats") also, *Makhai* ("Battles"), *Phonoi* ("Murders/Slaughterings"), *Androctasiai* ("Manslaughters"), *Neikea* ("Quarrels"), *Pseudea* ("Lies/Falsehoods"), *Amphillogiai* ("Disputes"), *Dysnomia* ("Lawlessness") and *Ate* ("Ruin/Folly"), all of one nature, and *Horkos* ("Oath") who most troubles men upon earth when anyone wilfully swears a false oath.

Strife appears in Homer's *Iliad*, Book IV, equated with *Enyo* as the sister of *Ares* and so presumably daughter of *Zeus* and *Hera*.

Strife whose wrath is relentless, she is the sister and companion of murderous Ares, she who is only a little thing at the first, but thereafter grows until she strides on the earth with her head striking heaven. She then hurled down bitterness equally between both sides as she walked through the onslaught making men's pain heavier. She also has a son whom she named Strife.[10]

This crescendo-like timing between the onset and peak effect of Strife is a stunningly dynamic portrayal of fomenting struggle. Conflict frequently starts as something small and, unreconciled, grows until the process itself takes on a life of its own, even beyond the inciting event or difference of opinion.

The most famous – and notorious – tale of *Eris* recounts her initiation of the Trojan War, with a (golden) Apple of Discord (temptation?) to be awarded by Paris, the prince of Troy, to the most beautiful of three goddesses – *Hera*, *Athena* and *Aphrodite* (who promised him Helen of Sparta). His choice of *Aphrodite* (and therefore Helen) prompted the start of the Trojan War, hence temptation's association with strife.

Harmonia

Harmonia's origins are not as clear as those of *Eris*. According to one account, she is the daughter of *Ares* and *Aphrodite*; by another, the daughter of *Aphrodite* and *Hephaestos*. By yet another account, *Harmonia* was from Samothrace* and was the daughter of *Zeus* and *Elektra*. Finally, *Harmonia* is explained as closely allied to *Aphrodite Pandemos*, the love that unites all people, the personification of order and civic unity, corresponding to the Roman goddess Concordia.

As the daughter of *Ares* (Mars) and *Aphrodite* (Venus), she was probably destined to promote harmony. Her range was substantial – she presided over marital harmony as well as the actions of soldiers at war. Late Greek and Roman writers sometimes portrayed her as harmony in a more universal sense – a deity who presided over cosmic balance.

---

* A Greek island in the northern Aegean Sea.

***

Current thoughts about the effective management of such interpersonal conflicts include the principles of *emotional intelligence*, generally interpreted as the ability to identify and manage your own emotions and the emotions of others. *Empathetic intelligence*, mentioned previously, adds to this the ability to put oneself in the shoes of the other. In contrast, and as a subset, *emotional intelligence* is generally said to include three skills: *emotional awareness*; the ability to *harness emotions* and apply them to tasks like thinking and problem solving; and the ability to *manage emotions*, including regulating one's own emotions and cheering up or calming down other people – the provision of harmony. Although the term first appeared in a 1964 paper by Michael Beldoch, it gained popularity in the 1995 book by that title.[11] A 2010 meta-analysis published in *Medical Education* by Arora et al. evaluated metrics of emotional intelligence and found correlation with many of the Accreditation Council on Graduate Medical Education (ACGME)-defined competencies that modern medical curricula seek to develop in trainees.[12]

Conflict resolution in a dynamic situation requires leadership. Is harmony the same as leadership? It would be foolish to underestimate the importance of good old-fashioned knowledge and technical ability (especially for surgeons and anesthetists) in clinical medicine. However, emotional intelligence can also be considered a key driver of success and leadership.[13]

The dark side of emotional intelligence – indeed "Harmony" – is that it can become manipulative when intelligently applied and cunningly practiced. The dialectic of emotional intelligence can be identified in the speeches of Martin Luther King Jr. and Adolf Hitler – both knew how to be spellbinding speakers and match nuanced emotional delivery to their words.

This manipulation can become theater of Shakespearean proportion – and occasionally is, on the Operating Room stage.

References

1. Cochran A, Elder W. Effects of disruptive surgeon behavior in the operating room. *Am J Surg* 2015; 209: 65–70.
2. Jackson S. The role of stress in anaesthetists' health and well-being. *Acta Anaesthesiol Scand* 1999; 43: 583–602.

3. Katz J. Conflict and its resolution in the operating room. *J Clin Anesth* 2007; 19: 152–8.
4. Chang J, Sy T, Choi J. Team emotional intelligence and performance: interactive dynamics between leaders and members. *Small Group Res* 2012; 43: 75–104.
5. Baron R. Positive effects of conflict: a cognitive perspective. *Empl Responsib Rights J* 1991; 4: 25–36.
6. Jehn K. A multimethod examination of the benefits and detriments of intragroup conflict. *Administrative Science Quarterly*; 40: 256–282.
7. Goodwin D. *Team of Rivals.* New York, Simon and Schuster, 2005.
8. Hesiod. *The Homeric Hymns and Homerica: Works and Days.* Cambridge, MA, Harvard University Press, 1914, l. 11–24.
9. Hesiod. *The Homeric Hymns and Homerica: Theogony.* Cambridge, MA, Harvard University Press, 1914, l. 226–232.
10. Homer. *The Iliad (440–445).* Cambridge, MA, Harvard University Press, 1924.
11. Goleman D: *Emotional Intelligence (Anniversary Edition).* New York, Bantam, 2006.
12. Arora S, Ashrafian H, Davis R, Athanasiou T, Darzi A, Sevdalis N. Emotional intelligence in medicine: a systematic review through the context of the ACGME competencies. *Med Educ* 2010; 44: 749–64.
13. *On Emotional Intelligence.* Cambridge, MA, Harvard Business Review Press. 2015.

12
FEAR AND PANIC: *PHOBOS*

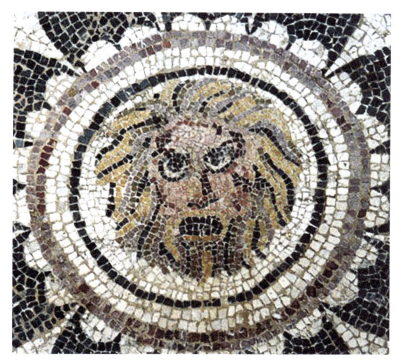

Fourth century CE mosaic with mask of *Phobos* (fear) within a radiating petal design. (Carole Raddato from Frankfurt, Germany, CC BY-SA 2.0, via Wikimedia Commons.)

Hours of boredom, moments of terror.

The above is a quote that seems to have much of its origin, or at least a burst of general use, describing trench warfare in World War I. There is a fondness among anesthesiologists and non-anesthesiologists for portraying the mindset of the anesthesiologist in this fashion as well. Often true of caricatures graphic or verbal, this quote captures more than a kernel of authenticity. As discussed by Gaba, Fish and Howard in their introduction to *Crisis Management in Anesthesiology*,[1] our role in the operating room, distinct from most specialties, is precisely this. Moreover, because of our proximity to the intimacies of patient care – direct dispensing and administration of some of the most potent medications known, the very person who rendered you unconscious and vulnerable is the one whose experience, skill and judgment you are exquisitely dependent upon. This is a heady environment in which to practice, the uncertainty of which (for the practitioner as well as the patient) has been discussed earlier.

***

Phobos ("fear") was the personification of fear. As the offspring of *Aphrodite* and *Ares*, he was "in the middle" of the conflict between love and war but became known as the companion of *Ares* in war, along with the sisters of *Ares*, *Enyo* and *Eris*, and his own brother, *Deimos*.

Those who worshipped *Phobos* often made violent, bloody sacrifices in his name. In the tragedy Seven Against Thebes by Aeschylus, the seven warriors slaughter a bull:

> Seven warriors (the leaders of the army of the Seven Against Thebes), fierce regiment-commanders, slaughtered a bull over a black shield (before the commencement of battle), and then touching the bull's gore with their hands they swore an oath by Ares, by Enyo, and by Phobos who delights in blood ...[2]

Warriors and heroes who worshipped *Phobos*, such as *Herakles* and *Agamemnon*, carried shields with depictions of *Phobos* on them in order to *invoke* terror and fear.

Hesiod described *Phobos* on the shield of *Herakles* as "staring backwards with eyes that glowed with fire. His mouth was full of teeth in a white row, fearful and daunting" and again later during a war scene as being "eager to plunge amidst the fighting men."[3] Additionally, *Phobos* was depicted as having a lion's or lion-like head:

> On the shield of Agamemnon is Phobos (Fear), who[se] head is a lion's ...[4]

According to Plutarch, Alexander the Great offered sacrifices to *Phobos* on the eve of the Battle of Gaugamela, hoping for Darius to be filled with fear. This was early psychological warfare through intimidation, often a successful tactic in the operating room as well. The brothers *Deimos* and *Phobos* were particularly worshiped in the city state of Sparta as they were the sons of *Ares*, the god of war. Spartan soldiers idolized *Phobos* because he symbolized discipline and consistency of the armed forces, striking fear into the hearts and minds of opponents.

There are many references within the Iliad to the roles *Phobos* and *Deimos* played on the battlefield:

> And he took up the man-enclosing elaborate stark shield *(of Herakles)*, a thing of splendour. There were ten circles of bronze upon it, and set about it were twenty knobs of tin, pale-shining, and in the very centre another knob of dark cobalt. And circled in the midst of all was the blank-eyed face of the Gorgo (Gorgon) with her stare of horror, and Deimos (Terror) was inscribed upon it, and Phobos (Fear).[5]

Homer spoke tersely and eloquently to the brothers' constant accompaniment of the god of war:

> So he [Ares] spoke, and ordered Deimos (Terror) and Phobos (Fear) to harness his horses, and himself got into his shining armour.[6]

Literally and figuratively, Fear and Terror served the God of War, Ares, well.

***

Emotional turmoil due to fear and panic impairs thinking and decision-making ability. Not surprisingly, participants in experimentally induced negative mood states perform worse than participants in positive mood states, however, both groups are outperformed by neutral mood reasoners.[7] Decision-making, so crucial to the practice of anesthesiology, is disrupted by such fear and anxiety. This well-recognized phenomenon in cognitive psychology is an emerging area of interest in neurobiology as well, with findings of suppression of spontaneous activity of prefrontal cortex neurons and weakening of encoding of task rules by dorsomedial prefrontal cortical neurons during decision-making.[8]

In a warring society (whether modern or Ancient), fear, like propaganda, was a tool to be utilized in order to wage a successful war. In a campaign of wills, as the operating room can occasionally become, striking fear or terror through intimidation, belittling, interpersonal struggle or exaggerations of petty perceptions, can be intimidating as well as demoralizing, yet it is unfortunately not uncommon, and often very effective. It is the basis for bullying. Understanding the context, and how to effectively apply emotional intelligence in order to neutralize it and continue forward with mental and emotional clarity is a crucial skill to develop. Moreover, the crucible of the operating room typically has at least two, and often three generations of practitioners in it, with varying levels of knowledge and experience as well as confidence, emotional intelligence and social skills.

Fearlessness is an unrealistic expectation when humans are hardwired for fear. But is it possible to place fear, and even terror, into a construct of "fear conditioning" whereby a neutral "charge" is assigned, rather than fear becoming the overwhelming basis for a response? Even if someone – a supervisor, a colleague, a consultant – tries to intimidate or belittle you, is anything really going to happen? Will you become diminished in any way by that action? Are you "actually" going to suffer? Is it a "real" threat? When the reality of the fear response is examined, there may be no threat at all in the fear/terror scenario. When neutralized and reframed, it then becomes possible to "flip" the fear and terror response to the positive side.

This technique, with better understanding not only of the psychological bases of the cognitive interference but also the biological bases of the amygdala's influence on executive function of the frontal cortex has been formally incorporated into military special operations training for Navy SEALs, for example. They adhere to four basic principles in attempting to tame the panic response and enhance decision-making ability in the face of fear:

1. *Goal setting* – in order to reset / enhance frontal lobe responsiveness, focusing on small, contemporaneous and incremental responses.
2. *Mental rehearsal* (sometimes known as visualization). Mental rehearsal and practice.
3. *Self-talk.* Mastering the attitude of "can do" rather than "can't do."*
4. *Arousal control* – focus on breathing, with long exhalation.

Most importantly as an antidote to fear, visualization is done to focus the mind on what can be controlled and the challenges to be identified. Self-talk with regard to mastering fear is about learning how to identify and change the conversation in your head, the interior monologue. This concept was expressed precisely by Shakespeare in Hamlet's response to Rosencrantz about Denmark: "There is nothing either good or bad, but thinking makes it so: to me it is a prison."[9]

The terrified target of the imposed fear needs to keep in mind that for the inflictor of fear, what is being gained from producing such fear is more than what he/she would gain from *not* producing the fear – or so it is thought. This is the true meaning of the backwards stare of *Phobos*. The perpetrator of the fear may be more afraid of failure than the victim. Then, this becomes the victim's most effective and best strategy. The price to be paid if the victim of fear and terror does *not* employ this strategy may be the avoidance of such situations and the eclipsing of long-term experience into a narrow window of recent belittling and intimidation. "Fear leads to anger ... anger leads to hate ... hate leads to suffering."† If occurring during medical care, the current patient as well as future patients may pay a price as well.

***

Fear was more poetically portrayed as relentless and unyielding in the *Iliad*:

---

* Reminiscent of the some of the sayings of the Star Wars character Yoda, including: "Fear leads to anger ... anger leads to hate ... hate leads to suffering" and "Do. Or do not. There is no try."
† Yoda, in Star Wars' *The Phantom Menace*, 1999.

As Ares is when he strides into battle and Phobos (Terror) goes on beside him, his beloved son, the powerful and dauntless, who frightens even the patient-hearted warrior: these two come out of Thrake‡ to encounter in arms the Ephyroi or the great-hearted Phlegyes (Phlegyans), but the two *will not listen to prayers from both sides, but give the glory to one side or the other.*[10]

Yet the allegorical truth about fear and terror portrayed by the Ancients was also revealed not by the infliction of their emotional burden on victims, but by their physical portrayal:

> The girl whose appearance in arms had revealed her as Minerva [Athena] was protected by two boys who were the comrades in arms of the battle-goddess, Terror (Terror) [Deimos] and Metus (Fear) [Phobos]; they pranced about with swords unsheathed.

Key to understanding the underlying weakness of terror and panic was this portrayal of Fear and Terror as boys, underscoring their immaturity. Because *Aphrodite* was their mother, *Phobos* and *Deimos* were also gods of the fear of loss. This important subtlety highlights the fundamental weakness of terror and fear as a strategic choice and exposes the vulnerability of *Phobos*.

References

1. Gaba D, Fish K. *Howard S: Crisis Management in Anesthesiology*. New York, Churchill Livingstone, 1994.
2. Aeschylus. *Works, Loeb Classical Library*. Cambridge, Harvard University Press, 1963, C5th BC, pp 41ff.
3. Hesiod. *Homeric Hymns, Epic Cycle, Homerica, Loeb Classical Library*. London, William Heinemann, 1914, pp 139 ff.
4. Pausanias. *Description of Greece, Loeb Classical Library*. Cambridge, MA, Harvard University Press, 1918.
5. Homer. *The Iliad*. Chicago, University of Chicago Press, 1951, l. 11. 36 ff.
6. Homer. *The Iliad*. Chicago, University of Chicago Press, 1951, l. 15; 119 ff.

---

‡ Thrace, an ancient country in the East Balkan Peninsula.

7. Jung N, Wranke C, Hamburger K, Knauff M. How emotions affect logical reasoning: evidence from experiments with mood manipulated participants, spiderphobics, and people with exam anxiety. *Experimental Psychology and Cognitive Science* 2014; 51: 570.
8. Park J, Wood J, Bondi C, Del Arco A, Moghaddam B. Anxiety evokes hypofrontality and disrupts rule-relevant encoding by dorsomedial prefrontal cortex neurons. *Jour Neurosci* 2016; 36: 3322–3335.
9. Shakespeare W. *Hamlet: A Tragedy in Five Acts.* New York, G.F. Nesbitt & Co, 1873.
10. Homer. *The Iliad.* Chicago, University of Chicago Press, 1951, pp 13, 298 ff.

13
LOVE: THE *EROTES*

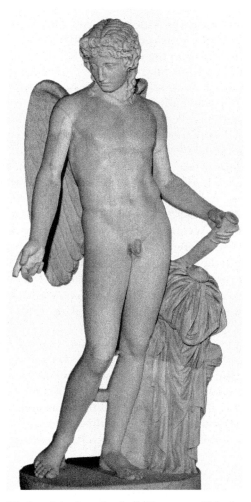

Eros Farnese. **National Archaeological Museum of Naples, Italy c. 2nd C. (Haiduc, public domain, via Wikimedia Commons.)**

DOI: 10.1201/9781003201328-17

Love is a complicated subject in mythology, as it is in the rest of life. *Eros*, as a single god, had several iterations, and the *Erotes*, as a group of gods, were associated with various facets of love, lust, desire and sex. The variously named *Erotes* were *Eros*, *Anteros*, *Hedylogos*, *Hermaphroditus*, *Himeros*, *Hymenaeus* and *Pothos*.

Eros

Eros, as understood contemporarily, is a creation of the later Greek poets. A more proper historical perspective on *Eros* recognizes three *Erotes* in the continuum of time: the *Eros* of creation, the *Eros* of philosophers and the *Eros* of the erotic poets. The last, with which we are most familiar because of the playfully sensual and frequently mischievous antics of the god, are generally not part of the ancient religious belief of the Greeks.

Hesiod (ca. 750–650 BCE) first represented *Eros* as a primordial deity who emerged self-born at the beginning of time. This early iteration made *Eros* one of the *fundamental forces in the formation of the world*, since he was the *uniting power of love*, which *brought order and harmony among the conflicting elements of Chaos*. It was said by Aristotle (384–322 BCE) as well as Aristophanes (c. 446 – c. 386 BCE) that he sprang from the world's egg.* Likewise, Plato (c. 427 – c. 347 BCE) refers to *Eros* as the oldest of the gods.[1] It is in accordance with the cosmogonic *Eros* that he is described as a son of *Kronos* and *Ge (Gaia)*. Pausanias (c. 110 – c. 180 CE) suggested that he had no parentage and came into existence by himself.[2]

The story is eloquently told by Aristophanes the playwright:

> At the beginning there was only Khaos (Chaos, the Chasm), Nyx (Night), dark Erebos (Erebus, Darkness), and deep Tartaros (the Pit). Ge (Gaea, Earth), Aer (Air) and Ouranos (Uranus, Heaven) had no existence. Firstly, black-winged Nyx (Night) *laid a germless egg in the bosom of the infinite deeps of Erebos* (Darkness), and from this, after the revolution of long ages, sprang the graceful Eros [the *primordial* Eros] with

---

* A cosmological view, in numerous cultures, of the very beginning of the universe, or being, accomplished by "hatching" from a primordial "egg."

his glittering golden wings, swift as the whirlwinds of the tempest. He mated [or fertilised] in deep Tartaros (the Pit) with dark Khaos (Chaos) [Air], winged like himself, and thus hatched forth our race, which was the first to see the light. That of the Immortals did not exist until Eros had brought together all the ingredients of the world, and from their marriage Ouranos (Uranus, Heaven), Okeanos (Oceanus, the World-Stream), Ge (Gaea, Earth) and the imperishable race of blessed gods (theoi) sprang into being. Thus, our origin is very much older than that of the dwellers in Olympos. We are the offspring of Eros; there are a thousand proofs to show it.[3]

Only the later iterations of *Eros* represented him as the mischievous god of love which we popularly recognize today, known for shooting love-inducing darts from his golden bow. Eventually *Eros* was embellished by ancient poets and artists into a host of *Erotes* (Roman – *Cupides*).

The singular *Eros*, however, remained distinct. It was he who lit the flame of love in the hearts of the gods and men, armed with either a bow and arrows or a flaming torch. *Eros* was often portrayed as the disobedient but fiercely loyal child and companion of *Aphrodite*. With time and the succession of the procreative to mischievous *Eros*, sculptors preferred the image of the bow-armed boy. Other artists favored the figure of a winged putto† (cherub), representing both innocence and mischief.

Purity was not essential to *Eros'* quiver. As the son of *Aphrodite*, his mischievous interventions in the affairs of gods and mortals often caused illicit bonds of love to form. He was represented as a blindfolded child ("love is blind") by many later satirical poets. This contrasted with his portrayal in early Greek poetry and art as an adult male embodying sexual power. The diminutive god thus portrayed the neutralized threat of sexual power.

---

† A *putto* is a figure in a work of art depicted as a chubby male child, usually naked and sometimes winged. Originally limited to profane passions in symbolism, the *putto* came to represent the sacred cherub. In the Baroque period of art, the *putto* came to represent the omnipresence of God.

Eros as a Weapon – Flattery, Charm and Deception

Nonnus of Panopolis (4th to 5th century CE), the last great poet of Antiquity, related how *Zeus* implored *Eros* to help him recover his lightning bolts from the great monster *Typhoeus*:

> You also, Eros, primeval founder of fecund marriage, *bend your bow, and the universe is no longer adrift.* If all things come from you, friendly shepherd of life, draw one shot more and save all things. As fiery god, arm yourself against Typhon (Typhoeus), and *by your help let the fiery thunderbolts return to my hand.* All-vanquisher, strike one with your fire, and *may your charmed shot* catch one whom Kronion (Cronion, Zeus) did not defeat; and may he have madness from the mind-bewitching tune of Kadmos (Cadmus)‡, as much as I had passion for Europa's embrace.[5]

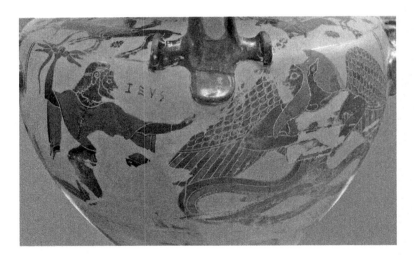

Zeus and *Typhoeus*. *Zeus* armed with a lightning bolt battles the winged, serpent-legged giant *Typhoeus*. Chalcidian black-figured hydria. (Staatliche Antikensammlungen, public domain, via Wikimedia Commons.)

---

‡ The founder and first king of Thebes. He was the first Greek hero and, alongside Perseus and Bellerophon, the greatest hero and slayer of monsters before the days of Herakles.

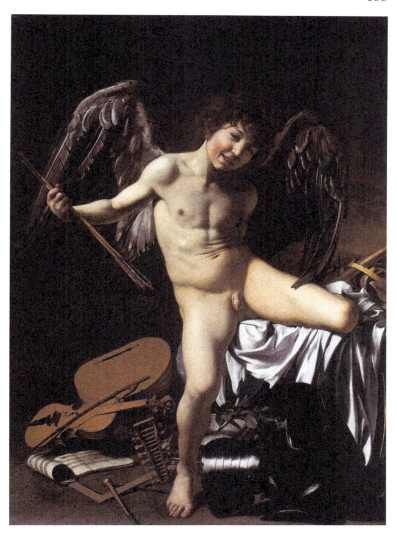

"Amor Vincit Omnia" (Love Conquers All) shows Amor, the Roman Cupid, with dark eagle wings. His ruddy face looks naughty. The painting illustrates the line from Virgil's Eclogues *Omnia vincit amor et nos cedamus amori* ("Love conquers all; let us all yield to love!").[4] (Caravaggio, public domain, via Wikimedia Commons.)

To think that as formidable a monster as *Typhoeus* could be conquered by using the power of Love! Nonnus expanded this theme with several additional examples, lending weight to what might otherwise be a coincidence. King Minos won a war against King Nisos of Megara with the help of the gods of love who made Nisos' daughter Skylla fall in love with Minos and betray her father:

> Kypris [Aphrodite] wore a gleaming helmet, when Peitho (Seduction) shook a brazen spear ... when the bridal swarm of *unwarlike Erotes* (Loves) shot their arrows in battle; I know how tender Pothos (Longing) sacked a city, when the Kydonian (Cydonian) trumpet blared against Nisos (Nisus) of Megara and his people, when brazen Ares shrank back for very shame, *when he saw his Phobos (Rout) and his Deimos (Terror) supporting the Erotes (Loves), when he beheld Aphrodite holding the buckler*§ *and Pothos (Desire) casting a lance, while daintyrobe Eros wrought a fairhair victory against the fighting men in arms.* For Skylla (Scylla), while her uncropt father was asleep, had cut off from his hair the purple cluster which had grown there from his birth, and by severing one tress from the sceptred head with her iron shears, sacked a whole city.[6]

Furthermore, *Beroe*, a nymph who was the daughter of *Aphrodite* and *Adonis*, was asked by *Dionysus* to surrender herself to love and desire, despite being destined to marry *Poseidon*:

> Obey the cestus girdle** born with the Paphian†† [Aphrodite], save yourself from the dangerous wrath of the bridal Erotes (Loves)! *Harsh are the Erotes when there's need, when they extract*

---

§ A small shield.
** The sash, or belt, of Aphrodite.
†† As a noun, one who engages in illicit love. Latin *paphius*, from Greek *paphios*, from *Paphos*, ancient city of Cyprus that was the center of worship of *Aphrodite*.

from women the penalty for love unfulfilled. Beware of the god's horrid anger, lest hot Love should afflict you in heavy wrath. Spare not your girdle, but attend Bakkhos (Bacchus) [Dionysos] both as comrade and bedfellow.[7]

Can Love actually disarm War? The Ancients certainly believed so at the wedding of Kadmos (Cadmus) and Harmonia:

> Her father [Ares] danced with joy for his girl, bare and stript of his armour, *a tame Ares!* And laid his right arm unweaponed about Aphrodite, while he sounded the spirit of the Erotes (Loves) on his wedding-trumpet answering the panspipes: he had shaken off from his helmet head the plumes of horsehair so familiar in the battlefield, and wreathed bloodless garlands about his hair, weaving a merry song for Eros (Love).[8]

Anteros

Anteros was the god of requited love, or love returned. At the time of the later iterations of *Eros*, he was the son of *Ares* and *Aphrodite*, given as a playmate to his brother *Eros*, who was lonely – the rationale being that love must be answered if it is to prosper. Describing the nature of requited love, Plato relates that it is the result of the great love for another person that is reciprocated. The lover, inspired by beauty, is filled with divine love and "filling the soul of the loved one with love in return." As a result, the loved one falls in love with the lover, though the love is only spoken of as friendship. They experience pain when the two are apart, and relief when they are together, the mirror image of the lover's feelings, or "counter-love."[9] *Anteros* was sometimes also the avenger of unrequited love.

Hedylogos

Hedylogos was the god of sweet-talk and flattery.

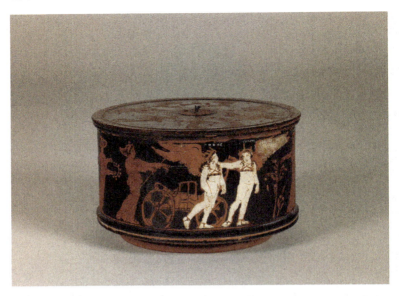

Red-figured pyxis (cosmetic box): this portion of the wall of the pyxis illustrates Aphrodite with attendants as she prepares to mount a chariot drawn by the Erotes – labeled Pothos and Hedylogos. British Museum. (ArchaiOptix, CC BY-SA 4.0 via Wikimedia Commons.)

Sweet-talk and flattery are often used in service of persuasion. *Honest* flattery is affirmative to the recipient and reinforces their self-image. *Exaggerated* flattery risks obsequiousness and borders on lying to the recipient, which they may or may not disavow. In the worst of possible worlds, not only does the recipient accept the (false) flattery, but incorporates it without denial, "embracing" the lie as truth. Indirect flattery, that flattery broadcast about someone to others, has a public relations feeling to it. For the recipient, it is a powerful way of enlarging one's audience. Flattery will get you everywhere. Note the hand on the shoulder technique utilized by *Hedylogos*.

In operating room social and professional discourse, flattery as persuasion should not be underestimated. When it is engaged in with love, it will be much less deceitful and importantly, will not be *perceived* as deceitful. It is a more graceful way of expressing and developing the art of persuasion when understood in the context of love rather than deceit.

Hermaphroditos

Hermaphroditos was once a handsome winged youth, like the other *Erotes*, but his form was merged with that of the Nymphe Salmakis in answer to her prayers that the two should never be apart. Metaphorically, it is perhaps the most extreme example of requited love.

> Hermaphroditos (Hermaphroditus), as he has been called, who was born of Hermes and Aphrodite and received a name which is a combination of those of both his parents. Some say that this Hermaphroditos is a god and appears at certain times among men, and that he is born with a physical body which is a combination of that of a man and that of a woman, in that he has a body which is beautiful and delicate like that of a woman, but has the masculine quality and vigour of a man. But there are some who declare that such creatures of two sexes are monstrosities, and coming rarely into the world as they do they have the quality of presaging the future, sometimes for evil and sometimes for good.[10]

This ultimate personification of requited love has its allegorical dialectic as well. Working in teams, as many do in health care, there is recognized value to collaborative models of diagnosis and intervention including predictability, reliability and consistent outcomes. The other pole of the dialectic occurs when independence of thought, opinion and intervention may become clouded and the value of independence both for the practitioner and the patient becomes painfully obvious. This not only extends to individuals but also to (specialty) groups that may share the same values within the group but may differ significantly between groups. Care must be taken to remain continuously aware of this form of self-love – and possible self-deception.

Himeros

Himeros was the god of sexual desire and longing who accompanied *Aphrodite* from the moment of her birth, He was first mentioned by Hesiod,[11] where he and *Eros* immediately appear as the companions of *Aphrodite*.

Himeros is omnipresent in celebrations of the *Muses*, the *Kharites*, the rites of *Aphrodite*, the revels of the *Satyrs*, and the merriment of *Bakkhos* (Bacchus), according to Hesiod, Pindar, Sappho and many others.

What place does the "god of sexual desire and longing" have in the context of professional development? It is a metaphor for passion driving an uncompromising level of engagement. "It's not just a job, it's an adventure" was a US Navy recruitment slogan in the early 1980s, and the same could apply to attracting anyone to a challenging career.

Hymenaios

Hymenaios was the god of the wedding ceremony who was supposed to attend every wedding. If he did not, then the marriage would supposedly prove disastrous, so the Greeks would run about calling his name aloud. He presided over many of the weddings in Greek mythology, for all the deities and their children.

The temporary marriage of surgeon and anesthesiologist is a tempting allegory, and while "true love" (i.e., mutual admiration), even for a short while could be an ideal, mutual respect, civility, and occasionally the ability to simply "get through it" on a professional basis, has to suffice. It may not, however, be totally inappropriate to think of the temporary union within the operating room in these terms, and along these dimensions – lest even the temporary marriage prove disastrous.

Pothos

Pothos was the god of passionate, sexual longing, yearning and desire. He was portrayed in a 4th century BCE krater as sprinkling his nectar of desire upon *Zeus* and *Europa* as *Zeus* carried her off to the sea. He was typically grouped together with the most commonly recognized three *Erotes* – *Eros*, *Himeros* and *Pothos*.

***

Through the stunningly creative literary strategy of dialogues, Plato has Socrates muse about the etymology of the names of the *Erotes* as he converses with Hermogenes and Cratylus:

> Sokrates (Socrates): Let us inquire what thought men had in giving them [the gods] their names ... The first men who

gave names [to the gods] were no ordinary persons, but high thinkers and great talkers ... [Of the Loves:] The name **himeros** (longing) was *given to the stream (rhous) which most draws the soul;* for because it flows with a rush (hiemenos) and with a desire for things and thus *draws the soul on through the impulse of its flowing, all this power gives it the name of himeros.* And the word **pothos** (yearning) signifies that *it pertains not to that which is present, but to that which is elsewhere (allothi pou) or absent,* and therefore the same feeling which is called himeros when its object is present, is called pothos when it is absent.

This is a sublime distinction between *object yearning* (for an object, person, task) you are facing and *abstract yearning* for that which you can't see in front of you.

He goes on:

And **erôs** (love) is so called because it *flows in (esrei) from without,* and this flowing is not inherent in him who has it, but is introduced through the eyes; for this reason it was in ancient times called esros, from esrein – for we used to employ omicron instead of omega – but now it is called erôs through the change of omicron to omega.[12]

The role of *Eros* was to *fill the recipient with love, not to kindle love within the recipient* – hence the arrow.

And here is where the relevance to professional comportment and teaching is most important. The filling of the recipient with the knowledge, joy and wisdom experienced by the teacher is a much more realistic goal than the hope, sometimes fulfilled and sometimes not, to kindle these values within the recipient. Medical teachers and senior mentors often try to ignite a passion that their students simply may not feel – at a particular time, or ever. But occasionally, one hears from former students or trainees, sometimes decades later, about how they have been influenced by something, even trivial, that they witnessed or heard you do. That is the most enduring example in medical teaching and training of the sustainability of the *Erotes* in fueling a passion for practice.

The prayer of Maimonides is probably second only to the Hippocratic Oath in its influence on Western medical ethics. Traditionally ascribed to Moses Maimonides (1135–1204), the great philosopher and codifier of Talmudic law, it says, in part,

> inspire me with love for my art and for Thy creatures. Do not allow thirst for profit, ambition for renown and admiration, to interfere with my profession, for these are the enemies of truth and of love for mankind and they can lead astray in the great task of attending to the welfare of Thy creatures. Preserve the strength of my body and of my soul that they ever be ready cheerfully to help and support rich and poor, good and bad, enemy as well as friend. In the sufferer let me see only the human being."[13]

As a teacher, I cannot more make you love what you do, but simply show you why *I* love what *I* do.

References

1. Plato. *Symposium. Oxford Approaches to Classical Literature.* Edited by Coleman K, Rutherford R. Oxford, Oxford University Press, 2004, pp 178, b.
2. Pausanias. *Description of Greece, Loeb Classical Library.* London, W. Heinemann, 1935, 9.27.1–3.
3. Aristophanes. *The Birds*, 4th edition. Oxford, Clarendon Press, C. 5th–4th BCE, l. 685 ff.
4. Virgil. *Eclogues, Loeb Classical Library.* Cambridge, MA, Harvard University Press, 1916, X, 69.
5. Panopolis No. *Dionysiaca, Loeb Classical Library.* Cambridge, MA, Harvard University Press, 1940, l. 400 ff.
6. Panopolis No. *Dionysiaca, Loeb Classical Library.* Cambridge, MA, Harvard University Press, 1940, 25, 150 ff.
7. Panopolis No. *Dionysiaca, Loeb Classical Library.* Cambridge, MA, Harvard University Press, 1940, 42, 378 ff.
8. Panopolis No. *Dionysiaca, Loeb Classical Library.* Cambridge, MA, Harvard University Press, 1940, 5, 88 ff.
9. Plato. *Phaedrus, Loeb Classical Library.* Cambridge, MA, Harvard University Press, 1937, 255d.
10. Siculus D. *Library of History, Loeb Classical Library.* Cambridge, MA, Harvard University Press, 2014.

11. Hesiod. *Theogony.* Cambridge, MA. Harvard University Press. 1914. l. 201.
12. Plato. *Cratylus, c 4th BCE*, trans. Lamb, WRM. 400 d and 419 e–420 b.
13. Friedenwald H. *The Jews and Medicine.* Baltimore, MD, Johns Hopkins Press, 1944.

Part IV

MORALITY

Morality and ethics are almost impossible to distinguish, at least etymologically. "Moral" comes from the Latin *mos* (L.: custom or habit) and is a translation of the Greek *ethos* (which means roughly the same thing). Morality is a set of customs and habits that shape how we think about how we should live or about what is a good human life. The moral rules of professional practice, for example, give meaning to the required knowledge and skills for medical practice. Among those *bona fide* morals particularly valued in medicine are truth, respect, justice, kindliness and self-control, personified as *Aletheia, Aedos, Dike, Philophrosyne* and *Sophrosyne*, respectively.

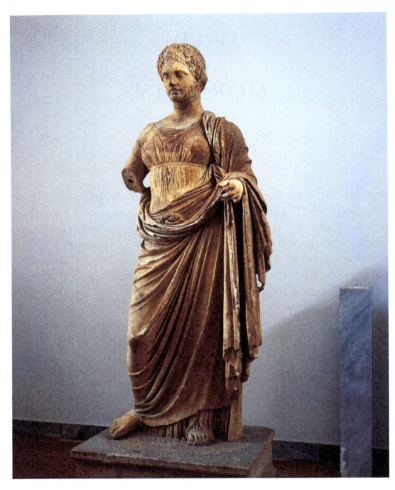

Themis, a Titaness, was the personification of divine order, fairness, law, natural law and custom. *Themis* means "divine law," literally "that which is put in place." She was the messenger of the first rules of conduct, established by the elder gods. As a divine voice (*themistes*) for justice, she instructed mankind in the fundamentals of justice and morality.

14
TRUTH AND LIES: *ALETHEIA* AND *PSEUDOLOGOS*

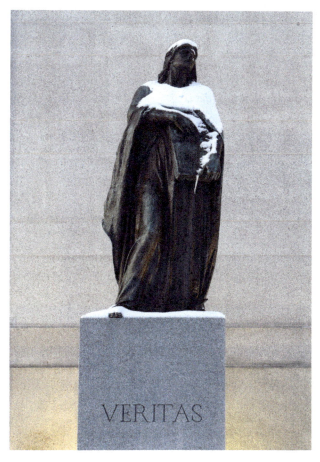

Statue of Truth outside the Supreme Court of Canada in Ottawa, Ontario.

DOI: 10.1201/9781003201328-19

Aletheia was the spirit of truth, truthfulness and sincerity, while *Pistis* was the spirit of honesty. In Roman mythology, *Aletheia* was known as *Veritas*. Variously translated as "unclosedness," "unconcealedness," "disclosure" or "truth," the literal meaning of *Aletheia* is "the state of not being hidden; the state of being evident." It is the opposite of *lethe*, which means "oblivion," "forgetfulness," or "concealment." Ironically, *lethe* was the basis for the initial name – Letheon – chosen by Dr. William T.G. Morton in late 1846 for his "new invention" – ether, ironically betraying his motivation for attempting to conceal the identity of the substance as sulfuric ether.

Distinct from *Aletheia*, *Pistis* was the spirit of trust, honesty and good faith. She was one of the good spirits to escape *Pandora*'s box and promptly fled back to heaven, abandoning mankind. Her Roman name was *Fides* (e.g., "bona fides") and her opposites were *Dolos* (Trickery), *Apate* (Deception) and the *Pseudologoi* (Lies).

The Pseudologoi were the personified spirits (*daimones*) of lies and falsehoods and were one of a host of malevolent spirits born of *Eris* (Strife).

***

It was Pindar who suggested that Truth was at the root of all virtue:

> Alatheia (Truth), who art the beginning of great virtue, keep my good-faith from stumbling against rough falsehood.[1]

Aesop suggested by parable that there is a time dimension to lies – that they become more prevalent with time:

> A man was journeying in the wilderness and he found Veritas/Aletheia (Truth) standing there all alone. He said to her, 'Ancient lady, why do you dwell here in the wilderness, leaving the city behind?' From the great depths of her wisdom, Veritas (Truth) replied, 'Among the people of old, lies were found among only a few, but now they have spread throughout all of human society!'[2]

A further parable from Aesop underscores a far more subtle point about truth:

Prometheus, that potter who gave shape to our new generation, decided one day to sculpt the form of Veritas (Truth) (Aletheia), using all his skill so that she would be able to regulate people's behaviour. As he was working, an unexpected summons from mighty Jupiter [Zeus] called him away. Prometheus left cunning Dolus (Trickery) in charge of his workshop ... Fired by ambition, Dolus used the time at his disposal to fashion with his sly fingers a figure of the same size and appearance as Veritas (Truth) [Aletheia] with identical features ... The master returned ... (and) ... was amazed at the similarity of the two statues and wanted it to seem as if all the credit were due to his own skill. Therefore, he put both statues in the kiln and when they had been thoroughly baked, he infused them both with life: *sacred Veritas (Truth) walked with measured steps, while her unfinished twin stood stuck in her tracks.* That forgery, that product of subterfuge, thus acquired the name of Mendacium* (Falsehood) [Pseudologos] ... every once in a while something that is false can start off successfully, but with time Veritas (Truth) is sure to prevail.[3]

***

Are transparency, honesty, and truth a continuum, or discontinuous points? Is all lying "black and white," or are there nuances to lying that serve greater purposes? Is all truth moral? Is all lying immoral?

"Transparency" has become a modern-day proxy for truth and honesty, but it is a term that ultimately is more anemic. Transparency in medical practice at the "system" risk management level incorporates the early reporting and analysis of adverse events, meeting with patients, families and health care professionals to provide explanations and support, and apologies and compensation for patients when the hospital and/or health care "system" is at fault. Such an approach is successful at the liability insurance level for conserving the costs of adverse effects of healthcare through communication and resolution programs (CRPs). At the institutional level, incident reports

---

* From which we get the adjective "mendacious" – untruthful, dishonest, deceitful, false, dissembling, insincere, disingenuous.

ideally increase, claims decrease, and legal costs as well as settlement amounts decrease as well. Transparency, as outlined in an editorial by Kachalia,[4] has the basic goals of improving accountability for safer systems, engaging clinicians in improvement efforts and engendering greater patient trust.

Transparency tells you *what* happened. Honesty tells you *why* it happened. The truth tells you how to examine the broader factors that contributed to its occurrence including the systems problems, motivational problems, individual problems, character problems, etc. They can overlap, to be sure, but there is much distance in the continuum from disclosing an error to examining the contributions to the error. Transparency is a meager substitute for truth and being honest is much harder than being transparent. Honesty means telling the truth, even when you haven't been asked a question.

Transparency puts every state employee's salary into a searchable database. Honesty means admitting that the highest-paid secretary is the boss's cousin. And integrity is not hiring the boss's cousin to begin with. For the individual as well as the group, integrity is the final goal.

Theories of Truth

Correspondence Theory

Correspondence theories emphasize that *true beliefs and true statements correspond to the actual state of affairs*. This type of theory stresses a relationship between thoughts or statements on one hand, and things or objects on the other. It is a traditional model, tracing its origins to ancient Greek philosophers such as Socrates, Plato and Aristotle. Thomas Aquinas (1225–1274) remarked "Veritas est adaequatio rei et intellectus" ("Truth is the adequation of things and intellect"), which is to say, a judgment is said to be true when it conforms to the external reality.

This is certainly closest to what most in medicine would accept as a validated and verifiable scientific basis of truth and what is most in keeping with Socratic, Platonic and Aristotelian notions about truth. The great Islamic physician Avicenna (Ibn Sina, 980–1037) also clearly subscribed to this theory when he defined truth as "What corresponds in the mind to what is outside it."[5]

Coherence Theory

For coherence theories, truth requires a proper fit of elements within an entire system. This contextual basis of truth, however, has not received widespread support because it does not lend itself well to empirical verification through observation. On the other hand, this theory closely conforms with our evolving political trend toward partisan truth.

Constructivist Theory

This theory is based in the notion that truth is constructed by social processes and is historically and culturally specific. It emphasizes the perception of truth rather than externally verifiable truth.

Consensus Theory

Truth is whatever is agreed upon by a specific group. During 2020 we have seen what this approach can lead to.

Deception

Deception is typically undertaken to hide the truth or promote a belief that is not true, usually for personal gain or other strategic advantage. Depending on the circumstances as well as the ultimate intent, a variety of tactics may be pursued to these ends – lies, equivocations, concealments, omissions, exaggerations, understatements and misinterpretations of the truth. All can be understood within the context of *accomplishing a goal that might not otherwise be attainable by telling the truth*: the avoidance of punishment, protection of possessions, maintenance of relationships or preservation of self-image.[6]

It is ironic that in the sacrosanct operating room the detection of deception can be so very obvious and its confrontation so challenging.

> How much longer until you are done?
> Why?
> Well, I'm trying to time the end of the anesthetic?
> 10 minutes.

... (45 minutes later) ...
I thought you said another 10 minutes?
Well, there were some technical issues.
Yeah, you decided to teach the medical student the proper way to close the skin.
Well, that's important ... you also teach medical students.
I thought you were going to give me an accurate estimate ... so you could get your next case started on time.

There are several levels of communication here. The possible offense taken by the surgeon after the inquiry may have resulted in a true estimate or a deliberate understatement as well as a misguided statement about technical issues and an off-putting challenge following even a minor confrontation – which was then rapidly concealed not by "what you said was a lie" but rather a self-image preservation response.

Many socially customary nonverbal cues that would be more readily detected behaviorally or by facial expressions are "masked" literally and figuratively by the garb and customs of the operating room. In addition, tension and fear, which typically result in changes in speech patterns and vocal pitch, can easily be an additional factor in the operating room. Eye contact, of course, is primarily dictated by the need to focus on the surgical field rather than between conversationalists, which often results in talking to the air.

Disguise, not in a costume sense but rather as a form of misleading information, is not uncommonly accepted as a mischievous component of interactions:

How much time will you need for this appendectomy?
Only 45 minutes.
(better book it for an hour and a half)

And:

Is the tube in? (the trachea)
Yes
Are you sure?
I think so.

There are statements that are transparent, statements that are honest, and statements that show integrity.

***

The Greek gods had an intriguingly amoral relationship with Truth and Lying, often preserving their power and accomplishing their desires through cunning, lying and deceit. *Zeus* often transformed himself into another person or animal in order subvert the power or take carnal advantage of another. *Zeus* constantly concealed his affairs with nymphs and mortals from *Hera* – the goddess of marriage.

Marriage quarrels among the gods were frequently based in lies of infidelity – King Tereus of Thrace lied to his wife, Procne, in order to sail to Athens and bring home Philomela, his wife's sister, whom he raped during the voyage. Once Procne found out – she then deceived Tereus and served him their son for dinner!

As amoral as the Gods could be, mortals, especially heroes, were held to a standard of obedience, while disobedience of a god brought immediate or eventual peril. The standard for Greek heroes, blessed with enhanced physical and mental strength was even higher because their honor and virtue were conferred through heroic accomplishments – like the 12 Labors of Herakles. Thus, a good life was achieved through the accomplishment of worthy deeds. The gods did not have to worry about paying their dues with worthy deeds.

Truth, Lies and Time

What Bridge(s), If Any, Exist between Truth and Lies?

If truth takes time, and most decisions in the operating room are made with the pressure of telescoped time, then much of the time that anesthesiologists spend is a calculus of certainty rather than certainty itself – or the management of uncertainty. (see Chapter 3) Relationships of long duration, for example, between surgeons and anesthesiologists who have worked together over years and sometimes decades, typically have much greater truth in communication than short-term relationships where uncertainty abounds because of lack of experience with each other as well as the procedures themselves.

In the Long Investment of Time Together, We Find Truth

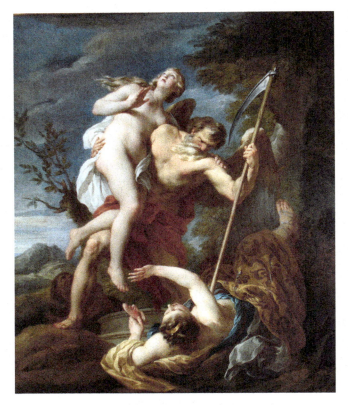

Time, Saving Truth from Falsehood and Envy. 1737. Time, holding a scythe, carries Truth, illuminated against a menacing background, while Lies and Envy lays, vulnerable, on the ground, holding a mask of deception in his left hand. François Lemoyne (1688–1737) (François Lemoyne, public domain, via Wikimedia Commons. The Wallace Collection.)

References

1. Pindar. *The Odes of Pindar*. London, William Heinemann, 1915. Fragment 205.
2. Babrius P. *Aesop's Fables*. Cambridge, MA, Harvard University Press, 1965, p 531.
3. Babrius P. *Aesop's Fables*. Cambridge, MA, Harvard University Press, 1965, p 530.

4. Kachalia A. Improving patient safety through transparency. *New England Journal of Medicine* 2013; 369: 1677–9.
5. Amin O. Influence of Muslim philosophy on the West. *Monthly Renaissance* 2007; 17: 11.
6. Buller D, Burgoon J. Interpersonal deception theory. *Communication Theory* 1996; 6: 203–42.

15
RESPECT: *AIDOS*

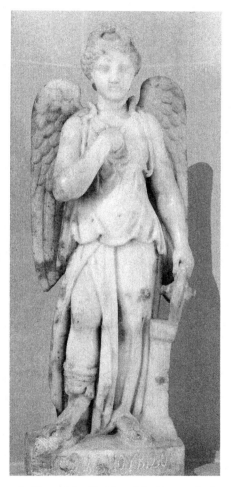

Nemesis, statue dedicated by Ptollanubis. Egypt, 2nd century CE. Her left hand holds the Wheel of Fortune, symbolizing her control of destiny. (Louvre Museum, public domain, via Wikimedia Commons.)

One of the striking things about the operating room is the uniformity of appearance of its personnel, almost a paean to egalitarianism. Everyone wears scrub clothes and other than name tags, there is really no way of visually identifying the role or rank of the individuals present. Yet once those roles are identified either overtly by nametags or covertly through behavior, the contrast is stark between informalities in the hallway and an almost ritualistic, highly choreographed and role-defined set of behaviors subscribed to not only in the moment but through literally centuries of indoctrination.

As a medical culture, we are currently deeply concerned about the idea of respect for persons, or more specifically, respect for patients as persons.[1] In the context of emotional support for trainees, this extends to medical students and house officers, clearly influencing their developing concepts of respect in conjunction with the health care team[2] and further contributing to improved team performance as a whole.[3]

***

Aidos (Aedos) was the goddess or personified spirit (*daimona*) of modesty, shame, reverence and respect. She was a companion of the goddess *Nemesis*. As a quality, *Aidos* was the feeling of shame which restrains men from doing wrong, while *Nemesis* was righteous indignation aroused by the sight of wicked men benefitting from good fortune earned without merit, committing crimes with apparent impunity. She was the punisher of hubristic boasts. Her name was derived from the Greek words *nemêsis* and *nemô*, meaning "dispenser of dues." As a personification of the moral reverence for law and the fear of committing a culpable action, *Nemesis* represented the development of conscience, and for this reason she is frequently accompanied by *Aidos* representing *Shame*, according to Hesiod.[4]

Euripides famously put it this way: "Nothing is shameful unless it seems that way to the person who does the act."[5] This utterly self-centered view of morality and self-respect discounts the influence of surrounding individuals and group judgment. Despite a distinctly narcissistic tone, the sentiment has endured and was repeated by Shakespeare's Hamlet two millennia later: "there's nothing either good or bad but thinking makes it so."

***

Indeed, the most common translation of the concept of *aidos* was not respect or modesty, but "shame." Why the apparent paradox? Across two millennia, the difference may be more apparent than real. In current thought we focus on how respect and modesty vs. shame and disgrace are almost mutually exclusive, yet the Ancients bound them irrefutably together. Characters in Greek literature, for example, refer to a personal sense of "aidos" as "what other people will say," representing at least one kind of shame. Moreover, "aidos" can be accompanied by blushing, or lowering one's eyes or the desire to hide. This is also where the component of modesty is suggested.

> Make his downy cheek as rosy as an apple, and, if possible, add a blush like that of Aidos (Aedos, Modesty).[6]

***

Of particular relevance to the development of conscience in medical practice, Bynum and Goodie explored the effects of shame associated with errors upon the wellness of learners. They described differences between shame and guilt in the health care learning environment and the importance of recognizing these emotions and their potential for occurring following a learner's error, explaining that shame involves a negative reaction to the worth of the self while guilt involves negative reactions to an action or behavior without implicating the value of the self. Misreading an X-ray is different than being an inadequate or bad doctor.[7] Whereas guilt is an emotion focused on a specific action, shame is a global feeling about oneself. Not only has everyone in medicine experienced this, but it is often recognized in the hidden curriculum as an essential part of training and a safeguard against hubris. Guilt is an emotion with a less pervasive effect on the individual. It allows the separation of the action from the self, holding it at arm's length and avoids the internalization that results from shame.[8] This distinction has been identified as a difference between "shame-cultures" and "guilt-cultures." What's at stake in this kind of shame-culture, then, is not a sense of responsibility in the face of a consciousness of wrongdoing, but a culturally specific demand for respect and honor.

Homer and Hesiod both addressed different kinds of shame and noted that shame depended on status and even class. They refer to the dialectic of *aidos*, or shame, and that it can be either a good or a bad thing, both harmful and beneficial. They also noted that it's something that tends to be harmful to the poor and beneficial to the noble or rich man. Euripides described it this way:

> And then there's shame, which has a double face: one, to be sure, is not an evil thing to possess; but there's the other shame, whose weight crushes whole households.
> *And if the good and the bad shame were easy to distinguish, the word describing them would not be the same.*[9]

while Hesiod advises:

> listen to right and do not foster violence; for violence is bad for a poor man. Even the prosperous cannot easily bear its burden, but is weighed down under it when he has fallen into delusion. The better path is to go by on the other side towards Justice; for Justice beats Outrage when she comes at length to the end of the race. But only when he has suffered does the fool learn this.[10]

***

What is it about shame that makes it *so* hard to tolerate? Why is it so intimately associated with respect and particularly self-respect in a Classical sense? And is a distinction between shame and guilt of any value in informing today's ethical and moral compass in medicine?

Along with embarrassment and guilt, shame is one of the emotions that motivates moral behavior. Current thinking suggests that shame is so devastating because it goes right to the core of a person's identity, making them feel exposed and inferior. It leads to avoidance and silence.[11] Yet many researchers claim – and medical educators operationalize – that shame has a positive role to play in social regulation as it inhibits antisocial behavior. Psychologists Trower and Gilbert, however, warn that fear of shame can result in "social anxiety, destructive conformity and unthinking deference."[12-14]

Competent doctors can therefore develop pathological anxiety.

Along the same pathway as shame and guilt, hubris (*Hybris*, as a spirit of insolence) added another dimension to the *Aidos – Nemesis* dialectic.

Pindar states:

> Hybris (Insolence) is the ruin of cities ... Never may shameless Hybris bring faction in her train and seize the company of citizens, when they have forgotten their courage.[15]

And finally, Aeschylus describes the most desirable of outcomes, equanimity and serenity:

> I have a timely word of advice: arrogance (*hybris*) is truly the child of impiety (*dyssebia*), but from health of soul comes happiness, dear to all, much prayed for.[16]

***

Why illustrate the concept of *Aidos* with *Nemesis*? Because the dialectic of respect, to the Ancients, was intimately associated with hubris and shame as its opposite defining quality. Self-respect was the issue – no self-respecting person could execute a shameful, indecent act. In the cultivation of that self-respect, respect for the other was a natural outgrowth. Now we focus on respect for the other. In accordance with the beliefs of the Ancients, respect for the other begins with self-respect and the avoidance of shameful, "indecent" acts.

The tension here is very significant. Humility often gets a chilly reception in medicine because it is sometimes seen as a sign of weak character. Yet humility remains deeply embedded in our culture. Humility was an important and heroic value of the ancient Greeks, who feared that excessive pride (*hybris*) would attract the savage vengeance of the inscrutable and remorseless gods. It is a peculiar kind of virtue. It requires that we do battle with some of our strongest and deepest inclinations, especially in medicine where advancement in academics and clinical medicine is predicated on achievement as well as self-promotion.

There is an additional peculiarity to humility. It is a virtue that ironically is constantly in danger of turning into its own opposite. As a result, what appears to be humility may very easily be, or become, something radically different from humility. The paradox is easily explained. As we become more accomplished in something, we tend to take pride in our advances and see our growing mastery, particularly when accompanied by the pleasure or approval of others, as a spur to further improvements.

To emphasize the point as an extreme – which is more important: having the appearance of virtue, or having the virtue itself? Which is more important, seeming or being? Aristotle had no doubt about the matter, but others (including modern achievers) are often less certain. Ideally, the virtuous leader should also take care to be known to be virtuous. This is an intriguing contrast to other virtues, such as courage, faith or perseverance. The more one possesses such a virtue, the more credible is one's possession of it in the eyes of others. Those who do increasingly courageous things are more and more evidently courageous.

Yet striving to appear humble is an instant disqualifier for anyone who actually wants to be humble. Witness Charles Dickens' character Uriah Heep, known for mendacious insincerity cloaked in the guise of humility.

***

The great heroes of Greek tragedy often exceeded decorum, shamelessly and disgracefully, with ambitions and vanities swollen beyond the limits that are granted to humankind. Such morality dramas served to define self-respect by making it an antidote to hubris, clearly a value to be deplored. The primary definition of respect, therefore, consisted of what it was NOT supposed to be. *Hybris* was a spirit or goddess of insolence, violence and outrageous behavior. In Roman mythology, the personification was *Petulantia*, identical to the Greek concept of hubris. *Aidos*, by being defined in a dyadic relationship with *Nemesis*, fulfilled the aspirational goal of respectful and modest behavior in the shadow of fear of shame and retribution. Respect was defined as the lack of disrespect.

Helping doctors to recognize and then address shame in themselves and their peers is thus vital for their well-being and patient safety. Understanding that shame can be experienced as discomfort highlighting a fault in self-image can guide trainees to become aware of their core values and use these as opportunities for self-development. Despite the repellent nature of the word, we really do need to talk about shame and its important role in forming a modern medical professional identity.

References

1. Beach M, Duggan P, Cassel C, Geller G. What does 'respect' mean? exploring the moral obligation of health professionals to respect patients. *J Gen Intern Med.* 2007; 22(5): 692–5.
2. Karnieli-Miller O, Taylor A, Cottingham A, Inui T, Vu T, Frankel R. Exploring the meaning of respect in medical student education: an analysis of student narratives. *J Gen Intern Med.* 2010; 25(12): 1309–14.
3. Riskin A, Erez A, Foulk T, et al. The impact of rudeness on medical team performance: a randomized trial. *Pediatrics.* 2015; 136(3): 487–95.
4. Hesiod. *Theogony. The Homeric Hymns and Homerica.* Cambridge, MA, Harvard University Press, 1914, l. 223.
5. d'Anjour A. *Shame and Guilt in Ancient Greece.* Presented at: New Imago Forum; 10 Sep 2016, Oxford. Accessed 1/23/21. www.armanddangour.com/2017/03/shame-and-guilt-in-ancient-greece/
6. Anacreon, Anacreontea, *Choral Lyric from Olympis to Alcman (Loeb Classical Library 143.* Campbell DA (trans). Fragment 17.
7. Bynum W, Goodie J. Shame, guilt, and the medical learner: ignored connections and why we should care. *Med Educ.* 2014;4 8: 1045–1105.
8. Cunningham W, Wilson H. Shame, guilt and the medical practitioner. *New Zealand Medical Journal* 2003; 116(1183): 1–5.
9. Kovacs D. *Euripides: Children of Heracles. Hippolytus. Andromache. Hecub. Kovacs D. vol 484.* Loeb Classical Library. Cambridge, MA, Harvard University Press, 1995, p 528.
10. Hesiod. *The Homeric Hymns and Homerica. Works and Days.* Evelyn-White H. Cambridge, MA, Harvard University Press, 1914.
11. Eisenberg N. Emotion, regulation, and moral development. *Ann Rev Psychol.* 2000; 51: 665–697.
12. Probyn E. *Blush: Faces of Shame.* Sydney, University of New South Wales Press, 2005.
13. de Hooge I, Bruegelman S, Zeelenburg M. Not so ugly after all; When shame acts as a commitment device. *J Pers Soc Psychol.* 2008; 95(4): 933–43.
14. Fessler D. Shame in two cultures: implications for evolutionary approaches. *J Cogn Cult.* 2004; 4(2): 207–62.
15. Pindar. *The Odes of Pindar.* Sandys J. Loeb Classical Library. William Heinemann, 1915.
16. Aeschylus. *Eumenides. Smyth H. vol 2.* Harvard University Press, 1926.

16
JUSTICE: *DIKE*

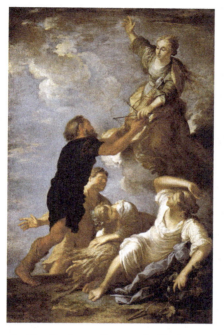

Astraea Leaves the Earth. According to Ovid, Astraea left the Earth, disgusted by the corruption at the end of the Iron Era.* She left her scales to the honest farmers.

---

* Mycenaean Greece collapsed around 1200 BCE, and Greece entered a period of turmoil sometimes called the Greek Dark Ages. Accompanied by famine, major cities (with the exception of Athens) were abandoned and people moved toward smaller, more pastoral groups focused on raising livestock. While Mycenaean Greece had been a literate society, the Greeks of the early Iron Age left no written record, a period that lasted roughly 300 years. By the late Iron Age, the Greek economy had recovered and Greece entered its "Classical" period.

"In seeing patients, physicians grapple with unemployment, housing instability, and food access; systemic racism, sexism, and LGBTQ rights; immigration reform, climate change, and violence. All of these issues profoundly – not tangentially – affect our patients' health."[1]

Policy-making bodies have been active recently in promulgating these advocacy points. The racial/ethnic disparities in health addressed in the Institute of Medicine report Unequal Treatment make it clear that the duty of a physician includes social responsibility and accountability toward the emotional, cultural and socioeconomic context of the patients he/she seeks to treat.[2] The Liaison Committee on Medical Education (LCME) has recently included cultural competency educational objectives necessary for medical school accreditation. The Centers for Disease Control and Prevention defines social determinants of health as "conditions in the places where people live, learn, work, and play" that affect their health outcomes and has as one of its Healthy People 2030 goals to "reduce the proportion of people who can't get medical care when they need it, and reduce the proportion of people who can't get prescription medicines when they need them." A 1998 article in the *Journal of Health Care for the Poor and Underserved* suggested the term "cultural humility" to replace "cultural competence," exchanging the notion of cultural mastery for a "lifelong commitment to self-reflection and self-critique" and acknowledgement of patient-physician imbalances.[3]

Conscience clauses† and provider refusal rules have brought the justice controversy in patient care into sharp focus. Examples include in vitro fertilization services to a same-sex couple or the provision of assisted suicide in a state in which it is legal. This protects the beliefs of the physician, who is nevertheless professionally and ethically obligated to refer the patient to someone from whom the care can be obtained. But a physician might also object to *treating a specific patient*, in which case it is not the

---

† A legal clause attached to laws that permit pharmacists, physicians, and/or other providers of health care *not* to provide certain medical services for reasons of religion or conscience. It can also involve parents withholding consent for particular treatments, such as reproductive care, for their children. In many cases, the clauses also permit health care providers to refuse to refer patients to unopposed providers.

treatment that is morally troubling but the patient him- or herself. Because the state licenses medical professionals and grants them sole authority to provide medical services to patients, physicians assume a positive duty to provide these treatments to the public.[4,5] Therefore, physicians who object to certain treatments have an ethical obligation to inform their patients about the availability of such (legal) medical services and to refer patients to other willing clinicians.

Physicians who object to treating certain patients, however, are a different matter entirely. Physicians who choose to help "acceptable" patients while refusing to care for others fail to live up to their ethical duty as doctors, and within the medical profession such behavior must be identified and actively discouraged. Such actions on the part of a health professional are a failure of justice in medical care.

Implicit bias[‡] has only recently begun to be addressed in the area of surgical, perioperative and anesthetic care, and the unconscious influences that are the underpinning of that care. Only a third of surgeons recognize that inequity contributes to worse surgical outcomes, higher postoperative mortality, and lower access to optimized anesthetic and pain management strategies.[6,7]

As anesthesiologists, our focus is typically on *how* we plan and conduct the anesthetic – anesthetic choices, hemodynamic management, attenuation of the stress response to surgery, choice of monitoring techniques – the pharmacology, physiology and anatomy issues. The justice perspective views *why* we do the case. Anesthesiologists play a critical role on the perioperative/surgical team and should take every opportunity to be advocates for justice in all forms for patients.

***

There were several goddesses and spirits of Justice – *Themis*, goddess of *divine justice*, to whom was born *Dike* (also known as *Dike Astraea* or simply *Astraea*), goddess of *human justice* and *Dikaiosyne*, the spirit of justice and righteousness. As the goddess of divine justice, *Themis* was the foundation of morality amongst

---

[‡] A preference for (or aversion to) a person or group of people, attitude towards people or stereotypy of people without conscious knowledge.

the gods. *Dike*, on the other hand, was to rule over human justice. Her opposite, in true dialectic form, was *Adikia* ("injustice"): in reliefs on the archaic Chest of Kypselos, an attractive *Dike* attacked an ugly *Adikia*, beating her with a stick shaped like a hammer.

Themis was a Titan, a daughter of *Ouranos* and *Gaea* and a deliverer of the first rules of conduct. Moreover, she was an early prophetess at the Oracle of Delphi, according to the Greek dramatist Aeschylus.[9] As a divine voice (*themistes*), she first instructed mankind in the primal laws of justice and morality, including piety, hospitality, good governance, conduct of assembly and offerings to the gods. As a prophetess, *Themis* foresaw some of the most famous prophecies such as the fall of the Titans (*Titanomachy*) where she prophesied that the war would not be won by brute strength and violence but by craft in gaining the upper hand. She also prophesied the death of the Giants (*Gigantomachy*).

According to Hesiod, *Dike* was a daughter of Zeus and Themis, and the sister of *Eunomia* and *Eirene*. The three sisters together were the *Horae*, the goddesses of the seasons and the natural portions of time. They presided over the revolutions of the heavenly constellations by which the year was measured, while their three sisters, the *Moirae* (the Fates) spun, measured and cut the thread of fate. *Dike* watched the deeds of man and approached *Zeus* whenever a judge violated justice. She was the enemy of all falsehood and the protectress of the wise administration of justice. *Hesychia*, the spirit of silence and tranquility of mind (and of interest to anesthesiologists, the handmaiden of *Hypnos*, or Sleep), was her daughter. The *Horae* were originally the personifications of nature in its different seasonal aspects, but in later times they were regarded as goddesses of order in general and natural justice. Of paramount importance to an agrarian society, "They bring and bestow ripeness, they come and go in accordance with the firm law of the periodicities of nature and of life." Kerenyi observed: "Hora means 'the correct moment'."[10]

Dike's name, $\Delta\iota\kappa\eta$, in Ancient Greek meant behavior in accordance with nature, without a moral connotation or limitation. Later, the name came to be more closely identified with "justice." She carried the Scales of Justice as a balance and wore a laurel wreath.§ *Dike* was often associated with *Astraea*, the goddess of innocence and purity. In Roman mythology, *Dike* was identified as *Justitia* who, in addition to the Greek iconography, was blindfolded, meaning that justice is impartial and objective. The first recorded appearance of the personified *Justice* occurred in Hesiod's Theogony where he described the forces of the universe as cosmic divinities and described *Dike* executing the law of judgments and sentencing together with her mother *Themis*. For Hesiod, Justice was at the center of religious and moral life, and embodied divine will. This portrayal of *Dike* and *Themis* contrasts with later views of justice as custom or law.

> Next he [Zeus] led away bright Themis (Divine Law) who bare the Horai (Horae, Seasons), and Eunomia (Good Order), Dike (Justice), and ... Eirene (Irene, Peace), who mind the works of mortal men, and the Moirai (Moirae, Fates) to whom wise Zeus gave the greatest honour, Klotho (Clotho), and Lakhesis, and Atropos who give mortal men evil and good to have.[11]

The Iliad and Odyssey of Homer are the earliest writing of justice as a concept by using the Greek words ("*dikē*") and ("*themis* ") designating "custom" or "behavior" in accordance with laws by human decree. Thus, *Themis/Dike* as *personae* represented the divine force that was higher than the laws written by man and promoted by decree. "Justice" was a force higher than "justice."

This notion of the development of the concepts of justice through time, from the divine to mankind to the spirit of justice and righteousness, *Themis, Dike* and *Dikaiosyne*, was reflected in the writings of the Ancients.

Fifth-century BCE playwrights saw *dike* in the cosmic sense as justice, often as punishment or retribution. All the characters in Aeschylus's *Oresteia* trilogy seek *dike* – "justice" – as punishment or revenge for previous wrongs. Through the fifth century, *dike* in

---

§ The laurel wreath symbolizes triumph. Apollo wore a laurel wreath on his head and wreaths were awarded to victors in athletic competitions, including the ancient Olympics. In Rome they were symbols of martial victory, crowning a successful commander during his triumph.

all its meanings – from judicial process to cosmic force – remains something external to human beings. *Dike* as justice personified was also developed by Sophocles and Euripides.

Solon (630–560 BCE) promoted *dike* – law-abiding conduct – as part of a general program of *eunomia* (good order, law and order). He also spoke of legislation as providing a "straight *dike*" (judicial process) for every Athenian thereby removing justice from divine law and into the realm of human law. *Dike* came to be seen in a new way – as universally applied equality. Heidegger, commenting on this migration from divine to human law, has pointed out that if this concept of *dike* is nonetheless accepted as the modern term "justice," i.e., judicial justice, it misses the original metaphysical sense of that ancient Greek word and may shortchange the original intent of symmetry with nature and the natural order of things.

***

There is a justice of rules and law, and then there is divine justice as virtue. The Ancients separated them as personifications but we would do well to remember, as medical professionals, that law and rules are the simplest form of justice and do not reach the level of virtue – only compliance. Perhaps Pope Francis (February 3, 2016) said it best: Human justice only limits evil, divine justice overcomes it.

References

1. Yerramilli P. *A Dangerous View: Why It's a Mistake for medical schools to Ignore Social Justice, STAT.* Boston, MA, Boston Globe, 2016.
2. Institute of Medicine. *Unequal Treatment: Confronting Racial and Ethnic Disparities in Health Care.* Washington, DC, The National Academies Press, 2003.
3. Tervalon M, Murray-Garcia J. Cultural humility versus cultural competence: a critical distinction in defining physician training outcomes in multicultural education. *J Health Care Poor and Underserved* 1998; 9: 117–25.
4. Cantor J. Conscientious objection gone awry: restoring selfless professionalism in medicine. *N Engl J Med* 2009; 360: 1484–5.
5. Charo R. The celestial fire of conscience: refusing to deliver medical care. *N Engl J Med* 2005; 352: 2471–3.

6. Britton B, Nagarajan N, Zogg C, Selvarajah S, Torain M, Salim A, et al. US surgeons' perceptions of racial/ethnic disparities in health care: a cross-sectional study. *JAMA Surgery.* 2016; 151: 582–4.
7. Butwick A, Blumenfeld Y, Brookfield K, Nelson L, Weiniger C. Racial and ethnic disparities in mode of anesthesia for cesarean delivery. *Anesth Analg* 2016; 122: 472–9.
8. McClain C, Stankey M. *Anesthesiology and Its Role in Functional Surgical Systems, ASA Monitor.* Chicago, IL, American Society of Anesthesiologists, 2021, pp 24–5.
9. Aeschylus. *Vol. 2. Eumenides.* Cambridge, MA, Harvard University Press, 1926.
10. Kerenyi K. *The Gods of the Greeks.* London, Thames & Hudson, 1951, p. 101 ff.
11. Hesiod. *Theogony, The Homeric Hymns and Homerica.* Cambridge, MA, Harvard University Press, 1914, l. 901 ff.

17
KINDLINESS: *PHILOPROSYNE*

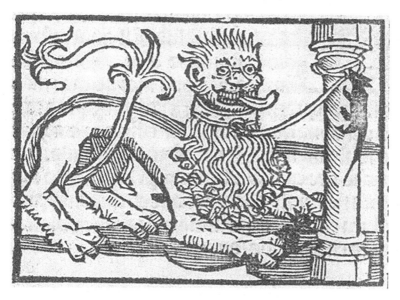

"The Lion and the Mouse" woodcut from the Spanish edition of Aesop's Fables. Ysopu hystoriado, 1521. (Unknown author, public domain, via Wikimedia Commons.)

A Lion lay asleep in the forest, his great head resting on his paws. A timid little Mouse came upon him unexpectedly, and in her fright and haste to get away, ran across the Lion's nose. Roused from his nap, the Lion laid his huge paw angrily on the tiny creature to kill her.

"Spare me!" begged the poor Mouse. "Please let me go and someday I will surely repay you."

The Lion was much amused to think that a Mouse could ever help him. But he was generous and finally let the Mouse go.

Some days later, while stalking his prey in the forest, the Lion was caught in the tangles of a hunter's net. Unable to free himself, he filled the forest with his angry roaring. The Mouse knew the voice and quickly found the Lion struggling in the net. Running to one of the great ropes that bound him, she gnawed it until it split apart, and soon the Lion was free.

"You laughed when I said I would repay you," said the Mouse. "Now you see that even a Mouse can help a Lion."

A kindness is never wasted.

(Aesop, c. 620–564 BCE)[1]

***

Philophrosyne was both a spirit (*daimona*) and a value. Etymologically, the suffix *-syne* serves to make a noun out of an adjective, while the prefix *-philo* means "loved" or "loving." "*Phros*" is related to "*phren*" representing "mind," so (very roughly) put together, *Philoprosyne*, as a value, suggests "*loving mindedness.*" As a spirit, *Philoprosyne* personified welcome, friendliness, and kindness. Her sisters were *Euthenia* (prosperity), *Eupheme* (words of good omen, praise, acclaims, shouts of triumph, and applause), and *Eucleia* (glory and good repute). Along with her sisters, she was regarded as a member of the younger *Kharites*.

This is an interesting distinction. The *Kharites* were divided by Hesiod into elder vs. younger *Kharites*. The elder *Kharites* – *Aglaia* (Beauty), *Euphrosyne* (Merriment) and *Thalia* (Good Cheer) – were the (more important) handmaidens of *Aphrodite* while the younger *Kharites* were frequently portrayed as attendants, of lesser importance. Among the younger *Kharites*, in addition to *Philphrosyne, Euthenia* and *Eupheme* were *Antheia* (goddess of floral decoration and adornment), *Eudaimonia* (goddess of happiness), *Paidia* (the goddess of play), *Pandaisia* (the goddess of banquets), and *Pannyachis* (the goddess of night festivities and parties). The younger *Kharites* were often portrayed as charming children, consigned to supportive roles accompanying *Aphrodite* as part of her Retinue, which included *Eros* and the *Erotes* and the *Horai*, goddesses of the seasons. Confusingly, the Homeric poems mention one *Kharis*, yet there are other Homeric references to an indefinite number. This may be a literary device to suggest that personified grace and beauty was divided into many beings to indicate the numerous ways in which beauty is manifested – one of which was kindness.

According to Horace and Pindar, the *Kharites* guided gracefulness and beauty in social life, fulfilled primarily by being in the service or attendance of other divinities. This was significant because it portrayed the essence of *real joy existing only when the individual gives up his own self and makes it his main object to afford pleasure to others through actions.* The grace accompanying these acts of kindness was their lack of hubris, as if to say the less beauty is fueled by ambition, the greater is its meaning. These are the values embodied in the *Kharites, who were important not by their singular impact but by their ubiquity and ever-presence in service to the gods.*

***

Compassion, empathy and kindness are often bundled together as essential to medical practice and patient interaction. It is important to parse these differences carefully. Kindness is distinctly different from due care and other acts that are required of professionals. *Kindness is a virtue* – not a requirement. A virtue is part of one's moral character while a duty implies an obligation to others, a rule of conduct.

Kindness is a personal rather than a professional value and highlights a historical tension in personalizing the practice of medicine. The notion that doctors should be detached from patients was endorsed by the iconic physician Sir William Osler: "This neutrality in witnessing human suffering gives him (the doctor) a special glimpse into the 'inner life' of patients."[2] An opposing view was offered in 1926 as the closing line of an address to Harvard Medical School students by Dr. Francis W. Peabody. In a subsequent seminal paper, Peabody said "One of the essential qualities of the clinician is interest in humanity, for the secret of the care of the patient is in caring for the patient."[3]

Contemporary medical practice continues to reflect a tension between these two concepts. In the rarified atmosphere of the tertiary care medical center where arcane yet accurate medical diagnoses can be made by the cognoscenti, many patients expect, even demand, a "House MD"* approach, where diagnosis is everything, even if a bafflingly elusive and tragic illness is diagnosed by a brilliant yet misanthropic doctor before the clock runs out. For television, this is dramatically appealing, narcissistically enticing and very unrealistic. Far less melodramatic (and therefore less appealing to commercial sponsors) is another narrative – comfort and kindness in addition to competent clinical care. Sadly, this former narrative has become commonplace, and even dominant, over the past 100 years. It is, moreover, a seductively "just in time" story we like to tell about ourselves.

The older narrative, which preceded this more recent revision for thousands of years, was common when doctors could do far less for patients. Today, rapidly lethal diseases and congenital malformations in childhood have changed into chronic disorders requiring a commitment to patients for whom management, mitigation, partnership and even negotiation are required in order to help them cope. This evolution has been acknowledged, in part, as the restitution vs. quest narrative in the domain of health care[4] and one of its principal requirements is a return to an old value – kindness.

The Restitution vs. Quest Narrative

In healthcare, **restitution** suggests that a once healthy body that has become ill will become healthy again. This is certainly what all patients hope for – the happy ending outcome – a cure. For many people with chronic conditions or illnesses, however, the reality is a chaotic journey through time where doctors cure, palliate, and also provide comfort and enhance coping. Many bonds are made along this journey. This is not the heroics of the misanthropic Dr. House who moves on after saving the patient's life. The patient is not the brief, passive recipient of care (as is usually the case with anesthesiologists). Trenchantly, the return to *status quo ante* is an axiomatic expectation in anesthesiology. It is all too easy for anesthesiologists – and others – to fall into the trap of arms-length engagement – our contact is intense but

---

* An American medical drama television series featuring a misanthropic medical genius performing diagnostic wizardry, which enables his cynicism, sarcasm and snark to be tolerated.

circumscribed, brief, full of uncertainty, and set within surgical and critical care. Vainly, it satisfies a heroic imago in the service of restitution.

A **quest narrative**, on the other hand, tells a story, often an epic saga, like the Odyssey, with Odysseus' journey back to his wife and son serving as the basis for the quest. When framing the quest, one describes his or her desire to do, see, experience or discover something. The quest narrative can be used effectively in many different contexts, including medical care – even in anesthesia practice. As anesthetists develop a more public voice and become increasingly recognized and remembered by patients, an emerging quest-oriented narrative can easily be envisioned.

What does this have to do with kindness? In the restitution narrative, doctors and others can view kindness as a "nice" but nonessential part of practice, something that can slow down and interfere with the efficient process of getting to a diagnosis and cure. At worst, kindness has been relegated to an attribute of losers rather than being an integral part of a doctor's duty to a patient. A paradigm shift toward kindness may require a change to a different narrative, a quest narrative, especially in light of our current trajectory. Safe, predictable, compliant, standardized and auditable medicine now involves pathways, guidelines and risk assessments. The technical and scientific elements of medicine outweigh the psycho-social care that is sometimes thought of as part of an outdated 'nostalgic professionalism'.[5]

With an estimated 250 percent increase in the number of people with long-term conditions over the next 40 years as well as the increasingly large fraction of the population achieving elderly status, the next phase of anesthesia care will be to create transitions to continuity. These transitions are already present in many anesthesiology subspecialties like pain management and palliative care and nascent in other areas such as critical care, obstetric, pediatric and cardiac anesthesia, especially in tertiary care centers where patients often return for repeated procedures and are well known by their anesthesia caretakers.

Kindness is not a gratuitous nicety in healthcare but rather the catalyst that makes scientific progress of most benefit to most people by promoting trust.[6] As for the concerns about the extra time it takes for kindness – the more work is motivated by kindness and the inevitable attentiveness and attunement it brings to patients' needs, the more it is likely to be effective, efficient and "right the first time." It also cements relationships between patients and their health care providers which is not only the right thing to do ethically but ultimately makes prudent sense with regard to risk management.

In recognition of these kindness dividends, efforts have been made to develop and document the "teachability" of kindness.[7] Ironically, this pedagogical approach to a more fundamental challenge may actually serve to avoid the issue rather than confront it. Rather than a skill to be acquired with practice or in the simulator, kindness, like background radiation, should be omnipresent. It is not simply a behavior that can be practiced or refreshed, but a hard-wired virtue.

Where might the deepest reservoirs of compassionate and kindly care exist in the cadre of medical professionals? There seems to be a difference in compassionate care through the aging spectrum – more junior physicians report greater barriers to compassion. Although many physicians enter medicine with a profound desire to help and care for others, there may be factors contributing to the erosion of this desire that should be identified. Moreover, within the pantheon of medical specialties, psychiatry might offer clues – working in teams, minimal distractions, frequent self-reflection, and practicing with emphasis on the therapeutic relationship. All of these may enhance medical compassion, and enhance the ability of an individual practitioner to preserve compassionate or kindly practice as an individual.[8] Anesthesiologists and other specialists stand to benefit, inasmuch as recent evidence with a simulated preoperative evaluation suggests anesthesia residents have variable as well as flawed recognition of patient cues, responsiveness to patient cues, pain management, and patient interactions.[9]

We care more about people who are close to us because kindness grows with familiarity. Because of this, continuity of care, a cornerstone of general practitioners for eons, needs to be built into specialty practices and health care systems. This is particularly challenging for anesthesiologists, yet solutions exist. One area of focus (at the single anesthetic encounter level) is the preoperative and postoperative visit. With current practice emphasizing efficiency and throughput, however, the person performing the preoperative evaluation is often in a preoperative clinic and will probably not be the patient's anesthesiologist. Moreover, these visits are days before the scheduled procedure, and because of the fluidity of the surgical schedule, assignments for clinical care are typically finalized the afternoon prior to surgery. Finally, many patients will be amnesic, especially if our medications like midazolam have done their job correctly, so patients will often not remember their anesthesiologist even when they have had a conversation with him or her in the preop period or in the Post Anesthesia Care Unit. A very simple solution has been to give out business cards to families as they exit the hospital, or a brochure within which business cards for the surgeon, anesthesia team and nurses can be inserted.

We care more when we are involved with a whole person than an organ or a specific task. The increasing specialization of care may further undermine this need for continuity, particularly in the high technology and advanced critical care specialties. One specialist focuses on the heart, another the lungs, yet another the kidneys and so on. Nursing has become a mirror image, with different practitioners appearing at the bedside: one for washing, one for nutrition, another for dressings and another for drugs, and yet another to explain what is going on. Balint referred to this phenomenon as the "collusion of anonymity" in which no one takes overall responsibility for the person because each professional is only responsible for their organ or task of specialist interest.[10]

***

Over 2000 years ago, Plato (428–347 BCE) described two types of doctors.

> For doctors, as I may remind you, some have a gentler, others a ruder method of cure. The slave doctors run about and cure the slaves ... practitioners of this sort never talk to their patients individually or let them talk about their individual complaints. But the other doctor who is a freeman, attends and practices upon freemen; and he carries his enquiries far back, and goes into the nature of the disorder; he enters into discourse with the patient and with his friends, and is at once getting information from the sick man.[11]

Plato's doctors, with their vastly different levels of engagement, are recognizable in our hospitals and communities today. Even Stoics, known as notoriously resilient, described the attachment of the self to others as circles of *oikesosis* (connection, affinity, affiliation) gradually radiating outwards like the ripples on a pond to eventually include all humanity. The Stoic philosopher Porphyry stated that *oikeiôsis* was the beginning of justice.[12] We depend on each other not just for survival but for human flourishing, both living and doing well, a fulfilling of our potential. Aristotle described this in the Nichomachaean Ethics as *eudaimonia* (one of the younger Kharites) – happiness.[13] This is the kindness–happiness connection, both for the patient *and* doctor. This extends the concept of *oikesosis* to *oikos* – family.[†]

There is also a legitimate self-serving aspect to being kind. Ballatt and Campling in their 2011 book *Intelligent Kindness: Reforming the Culture of Healthcare*,[14] summarize some of the evidence for the impact that kindness can have on our brains. For example, altruistic individuals show increased activity in the posterior superior temporal lobe when compared with less altruistic individuals. Individual acts of kindness release endorphins and oxytocin and create new neural connections. The significance for such plasticity of the brain is that altruism and kindness become self-authenticating. This positive reinforcement loop is stunning – kindness can become a self-reinforcing habit that requires less and less effort to exercise. Indeed, data from functional magnetic resonance imaging (*f*MRI) scans shows that even the act of *imagining* compassion and kindness activates the soothing and affiliation component of the emotional regulation system of the brain.[15] This may be the neurophysiological basis for why kindness is considered teachable – but it may need to be reinforced with periodic booster shots. Metaphysically, of course, it is reflected in the notion that self-interest and the interests of others are bound together – as it were, a part of the "natural order," much as in the personifications of the *Kharites* and the *Horai*, and in keeping with the philosophy of *oikesosis*.

---

† An extended "family," typically a social or socioeconomic group, often living in one house or part of one social unit (i.e., a farm or close but unrelated members of the same household).

Kindness requires action while compassion and empathy are thoughtful but passive states. Empathy in action is compassion.[7] An essential component of compassion is the feeling of interconnectedness with others, which naturally leads to engagement – a critical component of effective health care. In turn, being engaged leads to feelings of interconnectedness, compassion and satisfaction. Compassion and engagement are interrelated and self-reinforcing. Empathy, sympathy and compassion are often confused with each other and with a number of other processes involving sharing in another person's feelings. The key point here is that, if we are to be kind, then not only do we need to be sensitive to the suffering of others, but we also need to *make a constructive response* in such circumstances.

Is the word kindness more highly charged in medical practice than compassion, empathy or sympathy? The Ancient gods and spirits did not emphasize kindness as a virtue; it was not a large part of their theogony but was rather incorporated into the younger Kharites serving the gods. Kindness became part of mankind's routine vocabulary with the practice of medicine: kindness = compassion + action. In words often attributed to Hippocrates: "Cure sometimes, treat often, and comfort always."

References

1. Rinuccio D. *Libro del sabio et clarissimo fabulador Ysopu hystoriado et annotado.* Seville, Spain, 1521.
2. Osler W. *Aequanimitas.* New York, Nortop, 1963.
3. Peabody F. The care of the patient. *JAMA* 1927; 88: 876–82.
4. Frank A. *The Wounded Storyteller: Body, Illness and Ethics.* Chicago, University of Chicago Press, 1995.
5. Jeffrey D. A duty of kindness. *Journal of the Royal Society of Medicine* 2016; 109: 261–3.
6. Campling P. Reforming the culture of healthcare: the case for intelligent kindness. *BJPsych Bulletin* 2015; 39: 1–5.
7. Lantz-Gefroh V. *Making Medicine More Compassionate: It's Crucial—and It's Teachable, Scientific American Blog Network.* September 19, 2019.
8. Fernando III A, Consedine N. Barriers to medical compassion as a function of experience and specialization: psychiatry, pediatrics, internal medicine, surgery, and general practice. *Journal of Pain and Symptom Management* 2017; 53: 979–87.

9. Waisel D, Ruben M, Blanch-Hartigan D, Hall J, Meyer E, Blum R. Compassionate and clinical behavior of residents in a simulated informed consent encounter. *Anesthesiology* 2020; 132: 159–69.
10. Balint M. *The Doctor, His Patient and the Illness*. Oxford, International Universities Press, 1957.
11. Plato. *Laws Book IV*. Edited by Jowett B. New York, Dover Publications, 2006.
12. Richter D. *Cosmopolis: Imagining Community in Late Classical Athens and the Early Roman Empire*. Oxford, Oxford University Press, 2011.
13. Aristotle. *The Nichomachean Ethics*. Edited by Tredennick H. London, Penguin Books, 2004.
14. Ballatt J, Campling P. *Intelligent Kindness: Reforming the Culture of Healthcare*. London, RCPsych Publications, 2011.
15. Gilbert P, Choden P. *Mindful Compassion*. London, Robinson, 2013.

18
SELF-CONTROL: *SOPHROSYNE*

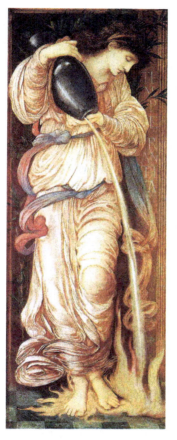

Temperantia. 1872 Edward Burne-Jones (1833–1898). (Edward Burne-Jones, public domain, via Wikimedia Commons.)

Temperantia (Temperance) was a companion painting to *Fides* and *Spes* (Faith and Hope). Some interpret it as an allegory of quenching the fires of passion, but this is only one of many meanings for the value *sophrosyne*.

DOI: 10.1201/9781003201328-23

Sophrosyne is an ancient Greek concept of excellence of character and soundness of mind. In the well-balanced individual, qualities such as temperance, moderation, prudence, purity, decorum and self-control, follow.[1] There is no equivalent word in other languages. *Sophrosyne* is compounded from two Greek roots, *sophron* and *syne*. Adding "*syne*" to the end of an adjective turns that adjective into an abstract noun, so *sophron* (sound-minded) + *syne* = *sophrosyne* (soundminded-ness). (*Syne* works similarly to the English suffix "-ness"). S*ophron* ("sound-minded") is a compound of two words: *soos* and *phren*. *Soos* is from the adjective *saos* (safe, protected or healed.) It is the root of the words for "savior" (*soter*) and salvation or safety (*soteria* – see Chapter 4). *Phren* in this context means "mind" but its Archaic use actually dates back to Hippocrates, for whom it designated the diaphragm.

The explanation for this apparently egregious inaccuracy when examined through 21st century eyes was discussed extensively by Plato, who located the soul within the thorax and thereby explained the role of the *phrenes*, or midriff:

> That part of the soul, then, which partakes of courage and spirit (*thymos*), since it is a lover of victory (*philonikos*), they planted more near to the head, between the midriff (*phrenes*) and the neck, in order that it might hearken to the reason, and, in conjunction therewith, might forcibly subdue the tribe of the desires whensoever they should utterly refuse to yield willing obedience to the word of command from the citadel of reason.[2]

Homer considered the *phren* to be the chest cavity itself. From the *Iliad*:

> But Patroclus in turn rushed on with the bronze, and not in vain did the shaft speed from his hand, but smote his foe where the midriff (*phrenes*) is set close about the throbbing heart.[3]

For Homeric heroes, this heated gas under pressure, the *thymos*, was not simply an emotion, but life itself. Its loss was death. The *phren*, or mind, was the organ of protection and control of this lifeforce, channeling its drive and energy in desirable directions. The *thymos* is the fuel of striving, but it always threatens to break out in competitive strife. It is the source of courage and the pursuit of honor. The *phren* controls the *thymos* by either venting it appropriately or dampening it through the cooling effect of the lungs. (Courage and moderation press against each other like force and counterforce – another dialectic.) *Phren* was usually written in the plural (*phrenes*) because it included the two lungs. Because of its influence over the passions, it became functionally equivalent to our understanding of "mind." For Homeric man, the mind of a human being was in his chest, because that's where the anger and passion were! *Sophrosyne* was therefore the spirit of moderation, self-control, temperance, restraint, and discretion – soundmindedness. As a *daimona*, she was one of the good spirits to escape Pandora's box and abandoned mankind in her flight back to Olympos.

***

Disruptive behavior in medicine undermines collaboration, communication, morale and patient care. It robs co-workers of the time they need to devote to their jobs, whatever that job is. And, sadly, it says far more about the disruptor than his or her target. The term disruptive behavior was originally used to describe any inappropriate behavior, confrontation, or conflict ranging from verbal abuse to physical or sexual harassment that can potentially negatively impact patient care.[4] A few examples with co-workers:

1. You "yell at" or raise your voice to a nurse or other co-worker.
2. You threaten a hospital employee with having him or her fired.
3. You throw anything, anywhere in the presence of anybody, in the hospital.
4. If you are on-call and you yell at the nurse when he calls you at home
5. You throw a surgical instrument "in the direction of" an operating room nurse because she handed you the wrong one.
6. Bullying

Other unself-aware situations occur with patients:

1. Breaking bad news in a busy corridor in the presence of medical students, nursing staff and other patients
2. Delivering difficult news (e.g., a life-changing diagnosis) without showing empathy or ensuring there is appropriate support available for the patient
3. Using poor nonverbal communication (no eye contact, focusing on the computer screen or notes)
4. Speaking ambiguously or not explaining in plain language.

In disruption, *hubris* insulates the disruptor from the self-awareness needed to detect and guard against interpersonal harm. In the highly charged atmosphere of the operating room or other critical care areas, anger and accusation, particularly between co-workers of unequal power, quickly results in a preoccupation with the injury to self-worth, leading to a degradation of professional duty to the task and to the patient. While a one-time occurrence followed by an apology and a frank discussion of circumstances may serve to salve and repair the situation in order to enable a working relationship to resume, recurrences resulting in the label "disruptive physician" typically lead to hypervigilance on the part of co-workers looking for anything else you do wrong – and they will find it.

Many administrative and policy-level solutions have been implemented since the concept of "disruptive behavior" has been introduced, such as educating oneself (or having the institution implement a remediation program of education, guidance or professional counseling). This strategy frequently results in anger management training as conditional upon continued employment. Attorneys are typically involved at the institutional level in order to indemnify the institution and secondarily to counsel the disruptor. At the behavioral level (and some of the strategies involve cognitive behavioral therapy) lists of behaviors to be avoided are generated (like the behaviors above, but a longer list). Some of the behavioral training is directed towards how to respond to complaints in a neutral, non-accusatory tone when they do occur, or recur. But these "strategies" beg the issue when cast against values, or virtues, because *sophrosyne* gives much better guidance with a richer vocabulary than behavioral prescriptions or rules.

***

In Greek literature, as in Greek life, *sophrosyne* was a crucial virtue. Its first use in literature was when Agamemnon decided to take Queen Briseis away from *Akhilles* in the Iliad. Homer described Agamemnon as lacking *sophrosyne*. *Heraklitus*[*] stated: "*Sophrosyne* is the greatest virtue, and wisdom is speaking and acting the truth, paying heed *to the nature of things*." Themes connected with *sophrosyne* and hubris figure prominently in plays of Aeschylus, Sophocles and Euripides; they all recognized *sophrosyne* as a virtue. This dialectic illustrates that *hubris* is the opposite of *sophrosyne*, because it is anathema *to the natural order*.

Sophrosyne was an important topic for Plato and is the main subject of the dialogue Charmides. Plato's view of *sophrosyne* is related to *harmonia* (also see Chapter 11):

> *sophrosyne* is the harmonious moderation of the appetitive and spirited parts of the soul by the rational part.[5]

In *Republic*, Plato described *sophrosyne* as "the agreement of the passions that Reason should rule" thus endorsing executive function over emotional chaos. But there were additional shades to *sophrosyne*, strongly illustrative of Greek polysemy – a single word having many shades of meanings.[6] In archaic poetry elite classes referred to *sophrosyne* with regard to non-elite groups, who should possess the good sense to adhere to the status quo and refrain from social injustice or civil strife. Sparta seems to have been particularly associated with this view. The playwright Aeschylus used *sophrosyne* to encourage others to refrain from violent behavior and in exhorting women to refrain from excessive displays of emotion. In relation to slaves, *sophrosyne* had an authoritarian sense, to show obedience to one's master. Euripides used the term to describe "control of desire." Phaedra in Hippolytus was unable to be *sophron* in the sense of controlling her desire, so she killed herself – a response that was considered *sophron* by the playwright.

Herodotus the historian used *sophrosyne* to describe tyrants, suggesting that it is the quality they typically lack. Thucydides the historian used *sophrosyne* in the sense of acting in a manner

---

[*] A pre-Socratic philosopher also known as "Heraclitus The Obscure." He wrote a single work, *On Nature*, from which only fragments remain.

beneficial to the state – obedience. Aristophanes, the comedic playwright, used *sophrosyne* to describe the control of desire (sexual practices and social interaction), the practice of moderation in one's expenses and the value of quietism (restraint from the dirty business of politics) and minding one's own affairs.

While initially outlined in Plato's Republic, *sophrosyne* was also recognized by the Stoics, Cicero, St. Augustine and St. Thomas Aquinas, who consolidated the polysemy into the four cardinal virtues:

1. **Prudence**: the ability to discern the appropriate course of action to be taken in a given situation at the appropriate time.
2. **Justice**: fairness; the Greek word also meant righteousness
3. **Fortitude**: also known as courage: forbearance, strength, endurance, and the ability to confront fear, uncertainty and intimidation.
4. **Temperance**: also known as restraint, self-control, abstention, discretion, and moderation which Plato considered (as *Sōphrosynē*, sound-mindedness) to be the most important virtue.

Thus, this concept of self-restraint had a complex taxonomy – it was comported in accordance with one's social status (man, woman, boy, girl, slave) as well as in continuity from the self (internal restraint) to external references (masters, tyrants, the state).

In *Republic* the virtues of justice and *sophrosyne* are kept distinct, despite the fact that they are closely linked, by having justice mean "to take care of one's own affairs," whereas *sophrosyne* is reserved for a type of harmony by which the different classes of the state, and the different parts of the soul, agree on just what constitutes "one's own affairs." Plato links this with the traditional sense of *sophrosyne* as "being stronger than oneself."

References

1. North H. *Sophrosyne: Self-knowledge and Self-restraint in Greek Literature*. Ithaca, NY, Cornell University Press, 1966.
2. Plato. *Plato in Twelve Volumes*. Cambridge, MA, Harvard University Press, pp 69d–70d.

3. Homer. *The Iliad of Homer. Rendered into English Prose for the Use of Those Who Cannot Read the Original.* London, Longmans, Green and Co, 1898, p 481.
4. Rosenstein A, O'Daniel M. A survey of the impact of disruptive behaviors and communication defects on patient safety. *Jt Comm J Qual Patient Saf* 2008; 34: 464–71.
5. Hyland D. *Plato and the Question of Beauty.* Bloomington and Indianapolis, Indiana University Press, 2008.
6. Rademaker A. *Sophrosyne and the Rhetoric of Self-Restraint: Polysemy & Persuasive Use of an Ancient Greek Value Term.* Denmark, Bill, 2004.

Part V

VOICE

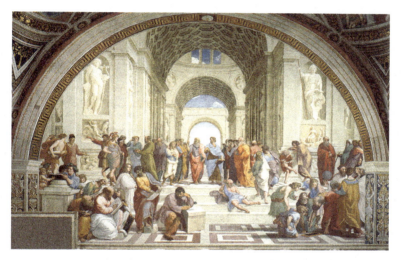

The School of Athens (1509–1511). Raffaello Sanzio da Urbino (Raphael, 1483–1520). Located in the Stanza della segnatura (Room of the Signatura), the first of four rooms in the Apostolic Palace (Vatican City) to be decorated by Raphael's frescoes. (Raphael, public domain, via Wikimedia Commons.)

Rhetoric, as described by Aristotle (384–322 BCE), was the "faculty of discovering in the particular case all the available means of persuasion." For the Greeks, rhetoric, or the art of public speaking, was first and foremost a means to persuade. Greek society relied on oral expression, which also included the ability to inform. This development followed several hundred years of transition from Greek monarchy to oligarchy and eventually, Greek democracy. This transition occurred from about 850–650

BCE, during the Homeric Period. The overthrow of Ceylon in 630 BCE by popular insurrection led to the codification of criminal laws into statutes of justice.

During the reign of Pericles (461–429 BCE) democracy advanced to the point where even poor citizens could serve on juries and make judgments in accordance with the established legal statutes. A popular legislative assembly reviewed all laws annually. Solon established the right for any Athenian citizen to propose or oppose a law during assembly. Athens became the center of western civilization – and with it came the need for public speaking. At this heady juncture, the enduring relationship of democracy and rhetoric were inextricably bound together.

19
CONSOLATION: *PAREGOROS*

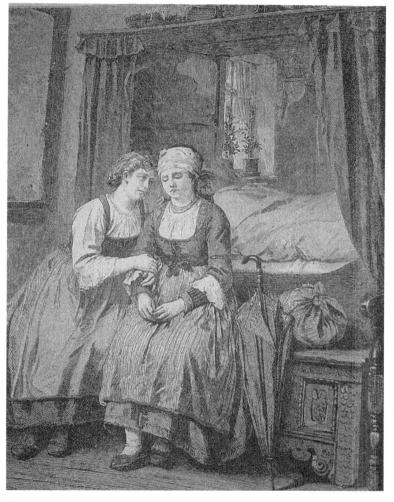

Consolation. A. Kindler (from l'illustration Européenne 1871). (loki11, public domain, via Wikimedia Commons.)

Before and after fundamental medicine offers diagnoses, drugs, and surgery to those who suffer, it should offer consolation. Consolation is a gift. Consolation comforts when loss occurs or is inevitable. This comfort may be one person's promise not to abandon another. Consolation may render loss more bearable by inviting some shift in belief about the point of living a life that includes suffering. Thus consolation implies a period of transition: a preparation for a time when the present suffering will have turned. Consolation promises that turning.[1]

***

Paregoron was the spirit daimona of consolation, comfort and soothing words. She was a companion of *Aphrodite*, the goddess of love, and *Peitho*, goddess of seductive words. Her statue, along with that of *Peitho*, stood in the temple of *Aphrodite* at Megara.

> After the sanctuary of Dionysus is a temple of Aphrodite, with an ivory image of Aphrodite surnamed Praxis (Action). This is the oldest object in the temple. There is also Persuasion and another goddess, whom they name Consoler, works of Praxiteles.[2]

Paregoric, a camphorated tincture of opium, is used to decrease stomach and intestinal movement, employed mainly as an antidiarrheal in children. Paregoric belongs to a class of drugs known as opioid analgesics, like morphine and opium.

Its etymology is interesting. As an Archaic adjective, it described the soothing or lessening of pain, and as an Archaic noun, it was a medicine that accomplishes the soothing or lessening of pain. The Latin *paregoricus* came from the Greek *parēgorikos*, which was derived from the verb *parēgoros* – speaking, consoling, soothing – compounded from *para* (on the side of) + *agora* (assembly).

In both ancient Greece and Rome, the *Consolatio* or consolatory oration was a ceremonial oration, used rhetorically as a public persuasion technique to comfort mourners at funerals. It was one of the most popular Classical rhetoric themes. As written works, Seneca the Younger (4 BCE–65 CE) produced the most recognizable examples of *Consolatio* in his three Consolations, *Ad Marciam* ("to Marcia"), *Ad Polybium* ("to Polybius") and *Ad Helviam Matrem* ("to the mother Helvia," Seneca's own mother). The *Consolatio* tradition is very broad, extending far beyond consolatory speeches to essays, poems and letters. This literary tradition flourished in antiquity, and its origins date back to the 5th century BCE. There were also scholarly *Consolatio* works on grief. These were often abstract, more third-person, essays. Orators in antiquity often delivered consolatory speeches to comfort mourners at funerals or in cases of public mourning. This oral and written *Consolatio* tradition continued through the Middle Ages and into the early modern era.

All *Consolatio* works are aimed at offering solace to allay the distress caused by the death of a loved one. A *Consolatio* often opened with "All must die." The most typical arguments characterizing the *Consolatio* were: "All must die; even the oldest must die; the youngest too must die, and this is as one with the death of the old."

One traditional delivery of the *Consolatio* deserves special mention, the use of *prosopopoeia*, when an author or speaker conveys the ongoing thoughts or opinions of a deceased person. A *prosopopoeia* is a rhetorical device in which a speaker or writer communicates to the audience by speaking as another person or object. The etymology is from the Greek roots *prósopon* "face, person," and *poiéin* "to make, to do;" it is one form of *personification* – the very basis for these essays! *Prosopopoeiae* are used to give an allegorical perspective on the action being described.

***

A doctor does not always heal and *cannot* always heal. Perhaps the hardest task knowing that he cannot be the deliverer of a hoped-for outcome is the provision of soothing consolation, so tersely put by the saying attributed to Hippocrates, "to heal sometimes, to comfort always."

The COVID-19 pandemic has brought a sharp acute focus on the role of the healthcare system in consolation. Unprecedented conditions – massive numbers of casualties, forced separations during a patient's final days, and denial of physical touch, final goodbyes, and traditional mourning rituals – pose threats to bereaved family members' mental health, leaving them vulnerable to intense and enduring psychological distress. The consolation needs are so immense, so overwhelming, that the sensibilities of the comforters are often clouded. Ways to communicate compassionately, assess risk for acute bereavement challenges, and refer to a mental health professional when indicated have been suggested based on research, clinical experience and common sense. A template for consolation has been offered in one notable review, and the principles bear repeating: **c**ommunicate compassionately, **a**ssess risk for acute bereavement challenges, **r**efer when appropriate, and **e**ducate about resources, altogether, recognized by the acronym CARE.[3]

As we learn more about the science of comfort and consolation not only in our own species but in others, a substantial neurobiological basis not only for the elaboration of oxytocin, the "love" hormone in the consoler, but an equivalent response in the consoled has been recognized. Consolation behaviors have the power to reduce stress hormones. Even the prairie vole, a social and monogamous rodent, will increase its grooming of his or her stressed partner with a commensurate rise in oxytocin levels for both partners. Interestingly, the unstressed partner matched the stressed partner in his or her stress hormone response, which suggests a neurobiological empathy mechanism. Moreover, the administration of an oxytocin antagonist blunts this consolation behavior.[4] These lines of discovery are strongly suggestive that compassionate care has a biological as well as psychological-emotional basis for reinforcement (also see Chapter 17).

For the Greeks, the public *Consolatio* remained among the most visible of oratorial obligations, perhaps none as famous as that of Pericles.

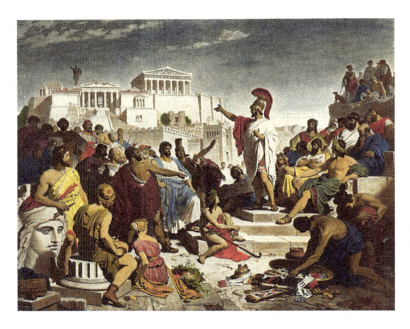

Pericles Gives the Funeral Speech. Philipp von Foltz (1852). (Philipp Foltz, public domain, via Wikimedia Commons.)

"Pericles's Funeral Oration" illustrates the public *Consolatio,* a famous speech from Thucydides' History of the Peloponnesian War.[5] Pericles, an eminent Athenian politician, delivered the oration at the end of the first year of the Peloponnesian War (431–404 BCE) when both sides retreated for the winter, as a part of the annual public funeral for the war dead. Different from the usual Athenian funeral speeches, Pericles' inspirational speech was a eulogy for Athens itself. It glorified Athens' achievements and was designed to stir the spirits of a state still at war. For example, the *Proemium* (preface) of the speech, began with "I don't know how I can do him justice..." and then, in a specific order: (1) *Proemium* (preface), (2) praise of the dead in war, (3) the greatness of Athens, (4) praise for the military of Athens, (5) exhortation to the living, and Epilogue. Not dissimilar to inspirational eulogies delivered in contemporary times, and more vivid (the Ancients would have used "persuasive," in keeping with the purpose of rhetoric) than the templated conversation referred to above:

One of the most memorable and best delivered speeches in modern times that followed this outline almost exactly was President Ronald Reagan's 1986 eulogy for the Challenger space shuttle crew:

> Nineteen years ago, almost to the day, we lost three astronauts in a terrible accident on the ground. But we've never lost an astronaut in flight; we've never had a tragedy like this. And perhaps we've forgotten the courage it took for the crew of the shuttle; but they, the Challenger Seven, were aware of the dangers, but overcame them and did their jobs brilliantly ...
> ... For the families of the seven, we cannot bear, as you do, the full impact of this tragedy. But we feel the loss, and we're thinking about you so very much. Your loved ones were daring and brave, and they had that special grace, that special spirit that says, "Give me a challenge and I'll meet it with joy." They had a hunger to explore the universe and discover its truths. They wished to serve, and they did. They served all of us ...
> ... I know it is hard to understand, but sometimes painful things like this happen. It's all part of the process of exploration and discovery. It's all part of taking a chance and expanding man's horizons. The future doesn't belong to the

fainthearted; it belongs to the brave. The Challenger crew was pulling us into the future, and we'll continue to follow them. ...

... I want to add that I wish I could talk to every man and woman who works for NASA or who worked on this mission and tell them: "Your dedication and professionalism have moved and impressed us for decades. And we know of your anguish. We share it." ...

... The crew of the space shuttle Challenger honored us by the manner in which they lived their lives. We will never forget them, nor the last time we saw them, this morning, as they prepared for their journey and waved goodbye and "slipped the surly bonds of earth" to "touch the face of God."[6]

***

The "rules" of the *Consolatio* were followed by Lincoln in the Gettysburg Address, which has been analyzed by American Civil War scholars.[7,8] Lincoln's speech, like Pericles':

- Begins with an *acknowledgement of revered predecessors*: "Four score and seven years ago, our fathers brought forth upon this continent ..."
- Praises the *uniqueness of the State's commitment to democracy*: "a new nation, conceived in liberty and dedicated to the proposition that all men are created equal ... government of the people, by the people, and for the people ..."
- Addresses the *difficulties faced by a speaker on such an occasion*, "we cannot dedicate, we cannot consecrate, we cannot hallow this ground."
- *Exhorts the survivors to emulate the deeds of the dead*, "It is for us the living, rather, to be dedicated here to the great task remaining before us."
- *Contrasts words and deeds*, "The brave men, living and dead, who struggled here, have consecrated it, far above our poor power to add or detract ... The world will little note, nor long remember what we say here, but it can never forget what they did here."

***

In addition to the pragmatic convenience of a template when providing consolation, we would all do well to remember the foundational importance of the Classical principles of *Consolatio* or *Paregoros*, and that consolation has both a private and a public voice in medicine and is an essential component of finding one's voice in the care of the patient and family.

References

1. Frank A. *The Renewal of Generosity: Illness, Medicine, and How to Live*, 1 edition. Chicago, University of Chicago Press, 2004.
2. Pausanias. *Description of Greece*. Cambridge, MA, Harvard University Press, 1918.
3. Lichtenthal W, Roberts K, Prigerson H. Bereavement care in the wake of COVID-19: offering condolences and referrals. *Annals of Internal Medicine* 2020; 173: 833–5.
4. Burkett J, Andari E, Johnson Z, Curry D, de Waal F, Young L. Oxytocin-dependent consolation behavior in rodents. *Science* 2016; 351: 375–8.
5. Thucydides. *The History of the Peloponnesian War*. Edited by Imrie A, Widger D, Project Gutenberg, 2009.
6. Reagan R. *Explosion of the Space Shuttle Challenger Address to the Nation, NASA History Web*. Edited by Garber S, National Aeronautics and Space Administration, 1986.
7. Warren L. *Abraham Lincoln's Gettysburg Address: An Evaluation*. Columbus, OH, Charles E. Merrill Publishing Co, 1946.
8. Wills G. *Lincoln at Gettysburg*. New York, Simon and Schuster, 1992.

20

ELOQUENCE: *KALLIOPE*

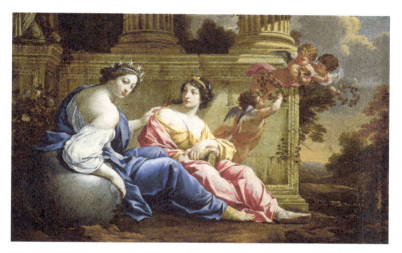

The Muses Urania and Calliope. C. 1634 Simon Vouet (1590–1649). (Simon Vouet, public domain, via Wikimedia Commons.)

The two female figures are *Urania* and *Kalliope*, two of the nine muses, goddesses who bestowed creative inspiration on practitioners of the arts and sciences. To the left, *Urania*, the muse of astronomy, is adorned with her crown of six stars and leans against a celestial globe. The second figure has a book in her lap inscribed "Odiss," Homer's Odyssey, which identifies her as *Kalliope*, muse of epic poetry.

***

Kalliope was the eldest of the Muses (*Mousai*), the goddesses of music, song and dance. She was also the goddess of eloquence, who bestowed her gift on kings and princes. In Classical times – when the Muses were assigned specific artistic imagos – *Kalliope* was named Muse of epic poetry and was portrayed holding a tablet and stylus or a scroll. In older art she holds a lyre (see front cover illustration). That this imago was hereditary was evident in Kalliope as the mother of *Orpheus*, citharist[*] and poet:

> Kalliope and Oiagros, though nominally it was Apollon, had as sons Linos, whom Herakles slew, and Orpheus, a professional citharist whose singing caused stones and trees to move.[1]

So great was consolation a portion of the oration corpus that *Kalliope* herself used this style to convey her eloquence at the funeral of *Akhilles*:

> To Thetis (*mother of Akhilles*) spake Kalliope, she in whose heart was steadfast wisdom throned: From lamentation, Thetis, now forbear, and do not, in the frenzy of thy grief for thy lost son, provoke to wrath the Lord of Gods and men. Lo, even sons of Zeus, the Thunder-king, have perished, overborne by evil fate. Immortal though I be, mine own son Orpheus died, whose magic song drew all the forest-trees to follow him, and every craggy rock and river-stream, and blasts of winds shrill-piping stormy-breathed, and birds that dart through air on rushing wings. Yet I endured mine heavy sorrow: Gods ought not with anguished grief to vex their souls. Therefore make end of sorrowstricken wail for thy brave child; for to the sons of earth minstrels shall chant his glory and his might, by mine and by my sisters' inspiration, unto the end of time. Let not thy soul be crushed by dark grief, nor do thou lament like those frail mortal women. Know'st thou not that round all men which dwell upon the earth hovereth irresistible deadly Aisa (Fate), who recks[†] not even of the Gods? Such power she only hath for heritage. Yea, she soon shall destroy gold-wealthy Priamos' town (*the city of Troy, of which Priam was king*), and Trojans many and Argives (citizens of Argos) doom to

---

[*] A citharode or citharist, was a classical Greek professional performer/singer of the cithara (lyre), using the cithara to accompany their singing.

[†] To pay heed to something.

death, whomso she will. No God can stay her hand.' So in her wisdom spake Kalliope.[2]

The importance of eloquence to leadership was evidenced with the bestowing of eloquence by Kalliope upon princes and kings:

> Kalliope, who is the chiefest of them all (the Mousai), for she attends on worshipful princes: whomsoever of heaven-nourished princes the daughters of great Zeus honour, and behold him at his birth, they pour sweet dew upon his tongue, and from his lips flow gracious words. All the people look towards him while he settles causes with true judgements: and he, speaking surely, would soon make wise end even of a great quarrel; for therefore are there princes wise in heart, because when the people are being misguided in their assembly, they set right the matter again with ease, persuading them with gentle words. And when he passes through a gathering, they greet him as a god with gentle reverence, and he is conspicuous amongst the assembled: such is the holy gift of the Mousai to men.[3]

Though eloquence is often invested with the use of fancy words and the ability to speak without notes, it is much more about how to get a message to live in the minds of an audience. Stating one's case logically, accurately and meticulously often won't be enough. Eloquence was expounded upon by Aristotle (384–322 BCE) in Athens. He saw how often a weak argument could triumph in public debate while a far more sensible proposal was ignored, not because listeners were stupid but because of how large a role our emotions play in determining the way that people react to what is said and to who says it. Ironically, Aristotle wanted to give more honest people the same weapons as the crooked, who were consistently successful at deception as well as persuasion. He lamented when people of ill-intent would know how to touch the emotions, while serious, thoughtful people stuck to plain facts. He developed a philosophy of the art of eloquence in order to teach how best to speak in order to be truly heard.

***

Health care professionals often play leadership roles, as authorities in clinical medicine or other aspects of health care delivery, research, or public health initiatives, especially lately. Some provide health education lectures in the community while others become involved in advocacy, making presentations to lawmakers or regulatory bodies. Strong public speaking skills are an important asset in all of these endeavors.

As a clinician, regardless of practice location, one attends seminars, conferences, rounds and committee meetings where there are expectations for participation and sharing of approaches to patient care with peers, coworkers and trainees. If one becomes involved in research, conferences and lab team meetings as well as mentoring sessions will occupy a significant amount of time, along with presentations in front of an audience. Honing your public speaking skills can help you take on a leadership role successfully.

When should "basic training" in eloquence for public speaking begin? Many would suggest it's never too early. Much like learning a language or a musical instrument, becoming a good public speaker requires time and practice. The premedical years of college offer a great opportunity to work on this; earlier would likely be even better. Medical students find out early that their presentation skills are crucial throughout their medical school careers, particularly during their clinical rotations. Intern and resident trainees are quickly and occasionally unceremoniously educated about organized, clear and concise clinical presentations of patients and subsequent plans for treatments and their justification,

Regardless of the composition of the audience, humanize yourself. Especially as an invited speaker burdened with the perception of eminence, there is a temptation to try to emphasize our prestige and stress our seniority and authority – a strategy that may accomplish the opposite. The audience may avoid engaging with what we say because they suspect we are looking down on them. The eloquent tactic, therefore, is to underscore our common humanity. A common tactic – a self-deprecating joke or a confession of anxiety – indicates that we too are flawed, worried and put-upon.

These tactics have a strategic goal – persuasion, the goal of rhetoric. Some of the new and potentially unusual things we will say should not feel like they are being uttered from a deity but from someone the audience can sympathize and identify with. The need to come across as ordinary is never more important than when one isn't quite ordinary in a specific setting.

Aristotle emphasized eloquent persuasion as fundamental to rhetoric. Rather than sponge-like, we are often more like sieves as audience members. We retain little, are easily distracted and allow our emotions to overpower our intellect. The individuals in the audience as well as the audience as a collective may feel envy, fear and suspicion. Our sympathies are moved more by individual cases (very typically true in healthcare as case reports) than by abstract issues. It is not enough to be accurate, concise, logical and data driven. We need to do the trickier thing: *touch the chords of the heart.*

***

Some 2,400 years ago, Aristotle, the world's first and arguably one of the greatest authorities on the subject, taught, whether in private or in public, *we speak for one reason: to persuade.* That can be challenging, because many of us suffer from speech anxiety We've never been trained to think strategically about communication. According to Aristotle's teaching on persuasion, the art of eloquence is explained in terms that have nothing to do with conquering anxiety or learning to be confident, but rather with learning how people listen to us. His beliefs and teachings were simple. He believed the most persuasive people:

1. *Think about their audience, not about themselves.* In public or private, he taught, we speak for one reason: to persuade. Aside from the subject, the eloquent speaker must reflect on:
    Who will be listening?
    How many of them will there be?
    How old are they?
    What race and gender?
    What do they know about you and your topic?
    Why are they gathering to listen to you?
    How can you help them?
    What is the purpose of your talk?
    Are you seeking to entertain, inform or inspire?

2. *Make their audience happy.*

Every element of the presentation should demonstrate your awareness of what the audience cares about. For example, a COVID-19 vaccination presentation will be far more successful to many lay audiences if the speaker illustrates the social, family, and business aspects of more rapid acquisition of high vaccination rates in concrete terms – when can I see my parents, when can my children see their grandparents, when can my business be "crowded" again? Television news programs are good at this because they understand their audience.

3. *Speak in their audience's language.*

Understanding the "culture" of your audience in a narrow as well as broad sense is crucial to effective, credible eloquence. Does the audience consist of clinicians, research scientists, perhaps both? Does the audience need to "hear" different views on the same topic – a clinical presentation directed towards medical students, postgraduate trainees, or seasoned clinicians? And if the audience is mixed – how do you want to recognize its composition?

***

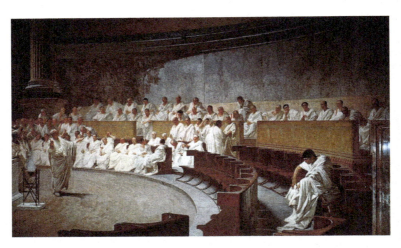

Cicero denounces Catiline. 1889 Cesare Maccari (1840–1919). (Cesare Maccari, public domain, via Wikimedia Commons.)

The discipline and eloquence of rhetoric were illustrated by Cicero in his four Orations against his political enemy, the charlatan Catiline, who conspired to murder Cicero and other key senators during an attempted coup d'état in Rome. Following four successive orations, the Senate issued a *senatus consultum ultimum*, a declaration of martial law and Cicero, as consul, was invested with absolute power. His opening remarks meted out his intention:

> When, O Catiline, do you mean to cease abusing our patience? How long is that madness of yours still to mock us? When is there to be an end of that unbridled audacity of yours, swaggering about as it does now?[4]

According to Petrus Paulus Vergerius (1370–1444), a wandering scholar and teacher in Italy and Northern Europe, who wrote the first syllabus[5] for a liberal arts education:

> I would indicate as the third main branch of study, Eloquence, which indeed holds a place of distinction amongst the refined Arts. By philosophy we learn the essential truth of things, which by eloquence we so exhibit in orderly adornment *as to bring conviction to differing minds*. And history provides the light of experience – a cumulative wisdom fit to supplement the force of reason and the persuasion of eloquence.

He continues, with a notable generational lament:

> and closely associated with these rudiments, the art of Disputation or Logical argument. The function of this is to enable us to discern fallacy from truth in discussion. Logic, indeed, as setting forth the true method of learning, is the guide to the acquisition of knowledge in whatever subject. *Rhetoric comes next, and is strictly speaking the formal study by which we attain the art of eloquence; which, as we have just stated, takes the third place amongst the studies specially important in public life*. It is now, indeed, fallen from its old renown and is well-nigh a lost art. In the Law Court, in the Council, in the popular Assembly, in exposition, in persuasion, in debate, eloquence finds no place nowadays: speed, brevity, homeliness are the only qualities desired. Oratory, in which our forefathers gained so great glory for themselves and for their language, is despised; but our youth, if they would earn the repute of true education, must emulate their ancestors in this accomplishment.

Aside from the perennial teacher's groan about superficiality in lieu of scholarship, there is a not-so-subtle cognitive science suggestion here – early experience with rhetoric may serve to enhance epistemological skills – it may not be that eloquence *follows* mastery of a corpus of knowledge, but rather that the development of eloquence as a formative skill *enhances* the acquisition and mastery of a corpus of knowledge. Hence – it's never too early to develop skills in public speaking.

Celsus (~ 25 BCE – 50 CE) writes of the eloquence of Hippocrates in the separation of medicine from (natural) philosophy:[6]

> we find that many who professed philosophy became expert in medicine, the most celebrated being Pythagoras, Empedocles and Democritus. But it was, as some believe, a pupil of the last, Hippocrates of Cos, a man first and foremost worthy to be remembered, notable both for professional skill *and for eloquence*, who separated this branch of learning from the study of philosophy.

Celsus also cautioned against glibness and ineffectiveness replacing effectiveness in medicine.

> it is possible to argue on either side, and so cleverness and fluency may get the best of it; *it is not, however, by eloquence but by remedies that diseases are treated. A man of few words who learns by practice to discern well, would make an altogether better practitioner than he who, unpracticed, over-cultivates his tongue.*

***

Audiences, whether a private conversation with an individual, public discourse with an audience, and even Zoom meeting audiences, want to be engaged with a speaker. Little formal teaching in medicine has been devoted to even the most rudimentary aspects of public speaking, let alone oratory or rhetoric. With *Paregoros* or *Consolatio* as a point of embarkation and *Kalliope* as the personification of Eloquence, our vocabulary for achieving this most sublime of requirements for promoting the art and science of medicine between and among our fellow human beings is enhanced.

References

1. Apollodorus. *The Library*. Volume 1. Cambridge, MA, Harvard University Press, 1921, 1.3.2.
2. Smyrnaeus Q. *The Fall of Troy*. Volume 3. Cambridge, MA, Loeb Classical Library, Harvard University Press, 1913, p 631.
3. Hesiod. *Theogony. The Homeric Hymns and Homerica*. Cambridge, MA, Harvard University Press, 1914, p 75HG.
4. Cicero M. *The Orations of Marcus Tullius Cicero*. Edited by Yonge C. London, Bohn, 1856.
5. Vergerius P. *De ingenues moribus et liberalibus studiis*. Edited by da Feltre V. Cambridge, Cambridge University Press, 1897, pp 2–104, 106–109.
6. Celsus. *De Medicina. Loeb Classical Library*. Cambridge, MA, Harvard University Press, 1971.

Part VI

ACTIONS

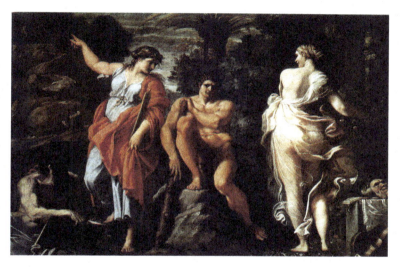

The Choice of Hercules, 1596. Annibale Carracci (1560–1609) Hercules is portrayed as uncertain about the choice between two destinies. The one on the right with a transparent dress represents Pleasure (*Kakia*) and shows him the flat road between playing cards, theatrical masks and musical instruments. The woman dressed on the left, on the other hand, represents Virtue (*Arete*) who shows him a tiring, narrow and uphill road, at the top of which, however, the winged horse Pegasus awaits him, which will lead him to glory and to heaven. (Annibale Carracci, public domain, via Wikimedia Commons.)

DOI: 10.1201/9781003201328-27

The Choice of Hercules by Carracci (1560–1609) is a graphic portrayal of Prodicus' (c. 465–395 BCE) essay Hercules at the Crossroads. This allegorical tale told of the young Hercules having to choose his path forward, confronted by Vice and Virtue. Vice's easy path will lead to pleasure and happiness while Virtue's harder path will lead to true and lasting satisfaction.

***

Herakles was a divine hero, and as both a hero and a god, he was immortal, invulnerable, and possessed godlike strength and stamina. The Labors of *Hercules* illustrated his heroic actions, although not all of his actions in subsequent events were heroic.

No seemingly intuitive action in the operating room is without knowledge, deep thought and judgement. Especially when life and death consequences have to be weighed, there is no room for partial effort. Inaction is often not an option and action within a context of uncertainty often occurs. Every action should spare no effort.

21
EFFORT AND LAZINESS: *HORMES* AND *AERGIA*

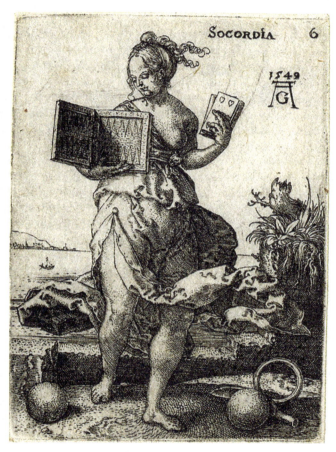

Engraving of Socordia (Carelessness) holding playing cards and a backgammon board. 1549. Heinrich Aldegrever (1502 – c. 1555). (Heinrich Aldegrever, public domain, via Wikimedia Commons.)

DOI: 10.1201/9781003201328-28

As one of the few extant graphic portrayals of the concept of laziness, *Socordia* (indolence, stupor, inertia) yields perhaps the most meaningful interpretation of this lack of engagement. Etymologically, it derives from sē- ("without") + cor ("heart as the seat of vitality"). So, this personification of a disinterested individual reflects the *Hormes – Aergia* dialectic. Full hearted versus no-hearted effort. Full engagement versus no engagement. Interest versus apathy.

***

Horme was the Greek female spirit personifying energetic activity, impulse, effort, eagerness and the setting of oneself in motion. In a warring society like Ancient Greece, a *hormê* was a violent forward movement – an assault or attack, especially the onrush of the battle. As a male, *Hormes* was also the personified spirit of effort, impulse and eagerness. *Hormes* was worshipped at Athens as the virtue of industrious effort, which was viewed by Pausanias as a moral component of piety:

> In the Athenian marketplace among the objects not generally known is an altar to Mercy, of all divinities the most useful in the life of mortals and in the vicissitudes of fortune but honored by the Athenians alone among the Greeks. And they are conspicuous not only for their humanity but also for their devotion to religion. They have an altar to Shamefastness, one to Rumor and one to Effort. It is quite obvious that those who excel in piety are correspondingly rewarded by good fortune.[1]

It is ironic when viewed contemporarily, but not surprising within the context of Ancient descriptions, that so little in writing or historical art is devoted to the value known as "effort." Modern usage ties the concept of effort to a general description of work, exertion or undertaking. Ancient descriptions were more contextualized – for example, the effort of battle, scholarly achievement, or public oration. It was the common thread of full-hearted engagement – effort defined by context – that permeated these disparate activities.

The opposite deity for both *Horme* and *Hormes* was *Aergia*, goddess of sloth and apathy, and the transliteration of the Latin *Socordia*. As a violation of piety, sloth was seen as a failure to utilize your gifts and talents, whereupon you become a burden when others are forced to do your work. Such a feckless individual, lacking character, eventually becomes a self-burden. This lassitude grows into a narcissistic rationale of being a prisoner of impossible constraints and an impossible life. Hopelessness and sulking color everything.

In Ancient allegory, the soul, under this influence of *Aergia*, enters the realm of *Hypnos*, the god of Sleep. *Hypnos* was the *daimon* of sleep and his realm resided within the recesses of the night (*Nyx*) – his mother, along with his brothers *Thanatos* (death) and *Oneiro* or *Morpheus* (dreams) (see Chapter 3). Succumbing to the values of *Aergia*, this soul fell into *accidia*.* [2,3] Viewed as a dialectic, *accidia* was the opposite of commitment, engagement, and love (see Chapter 13).

***

Hormesis, as a biological process, is characterized by a biphasic response to exposure to increasing amounts of a substance or condition. Within the hormetic zone, there is generally a favorable biological response to low exposures to toxins and other stressors.

It's use in relation to pharmacology can be traced back to a quote by Paracelsus: "All things are poison, and nothing is without poison; the dosage alone makes it so a thing is not a poison."[4] For this reason, the concept of *hormesis* holds a special place in the practice of anesthesia which – after all – is the therapeutic use of controlled dosing of poisons to interfere with the natural order of neurotransmission in order to produce a salutary result. The clinical practice of anesthesia requires a highly focused effort while anatomic and physiological transgressions conspire to challenge a human's existence, with the short- and long-term hope of curing disease and restoring function. Particularly with the use of some of the most potent pharmaceuticals known, the restoration of *status quo ante*, in some countries called reanimation, is the goal of this focused effort. The disruption of a natural

---

* *Accidia* or *Acedia* is a state of listlessness or torpor, of not caring. In Ancient Greece *acedia* originally meant indifference or carelessness. On the battlefield, Homer used it in the *Iliad* to contrast committed and indifferent treatment of a fallen comrade.

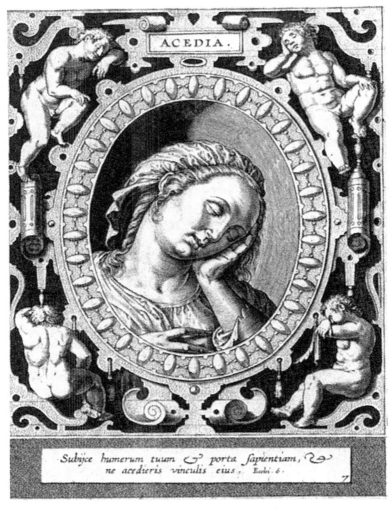

Acedia, engraving by Hieronymus Wierix (c. 1553–1619). *Acedia* is the personification of sloth (apathy and inactivity) as one of the seven deadly sins. (Hieronymus Wierix, public domain, via Wikimedia Commons.)

(neurotransmission) process is the very purpose of "anaisthesia" – a not-feeling pain (see Chapter 6).

***

There has been a growing awareness in anesthesiology among other critical care specialties of amplifying this concept in an attempt to mitigate biological injury. In biology, *hormesis* refers to adaptive responses of biological systems to moderate environmental or self-imposed challenges through which the system improves its functionality and/or tolerance to more severe challenges. This critical concept suggests a fertile avenue of research in, for example, acute lung injury (pre-conditioning for the blunting of inflammatory responses following acute lung injury), myocardial ischemia (ischemia-reperfusion injury), acute kidney injury and intestinal inflammation such as inflammatory bowel disease via boosting of adenosine levels in experimental colitis.

The concept of hormesis has much evolutionary precedent. For example, hormesis-based adaptations enabled organisms to survive and flourish in the presence of toxic metals. The solubilization of iron and copper in rocks results in the formation of ions (Fe^{2+} and Cu^+) that can be highly toxic to cells. During respiration (oxidative phosphorylation), cells generate hydrogen peroxide (H_2O_2) which, when reacting with Fe^{2+} or Cu^+ results in the generation of the hydroxyl free radical (OH^-), which can kill cells by damaging DNA, proteins, and membrane lipids. Very early in evolution, organisms evolved proteins to protect themselves against Fe^{2+} or Cu^+ toxicity. In addition, various iron- or copper-dependent enzymes evolved that used the redox properties of these elements to enhance their efficacy.[5]

The evolutionary "commitment" to biological effectiveness mirrors the effort-based, full-hearted requirement on the human scale to action. It is the full-hearted engagement required for ultimate success, which the Ancients as well as the Moderns recognize as Victory.

***

Perhaps the contemporary interpretation of action and laziness lies in the metaphor of the heart – half-hearted (*Socordia, Aergia*) and full-hearted (*Hormes*). This *is* the action of health care– not consisting so much of impulsive, flagrant activity but rather a depth of active commitment, engagement and focus brought to bear for the good of the patient – action of the mind, full-hearted, not half-hearted.

That level of commitment to the seven sections discussed in this series of essays – the human condition, qualities of practice, the emotions, morality, voice, actions and society – are the dimensions fulfilled at the highest level of practice. Commitment *is* the action, not battle, as it was in a warrior-state like Ancient Greece but the intellectual and humanitarian war of the care of our fellow humans.

References

1. Pausanias. *Description of Greece*. Vol. 1 Cambridge, MA, Harvard University Press, 1918, 1.17.1.
2. Homer. *Iliad*. *Book 14*. perseus.tufts.edu, line 427. Accessed 4/16/21.
3. Homer. *Iliad*. *Book 24*. perseus.tufts.edu, l ine 513. Accessed 4/16/21.
4. Paracelsus. Die dritte Defension wegen des Schreibens der neuen Rezepte: Septem Defensiones. *Darmstadt* 1538, p 510.
5. Calabrese E, Mattson M. How does hormesis impact biology, toxicology, and medicine? *Aging and Mechanisms of Disease* 2017 (epub date 15 September 2017). doi: 10.1038/s41514-017-0013-z.

22

VICTORY AND RETREAT: *NIKE* AND *PALIOXIS*

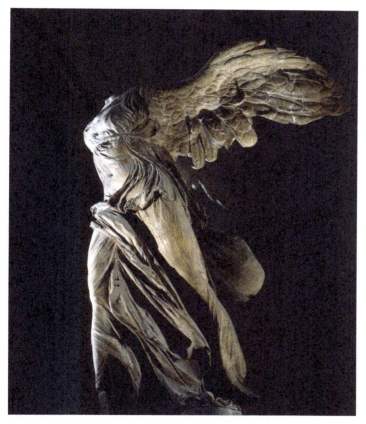

Nike. Winged Victory of Samothrace. c. 220–185 BCE. Three-quarter left view.

In comparison with the dearth of information about effort in the Ancient world, no vacuum exists celebrating victory (*Nike*) in

Greek society. As we have seen, the Greeks personified concepts such as Uncertainty, Safety, Pain, Disease and Scholarship as gods and spirits; *Nike* was one of the earliest of these incarnations. Her large wings enabled her to fly over the earth spreading news of victory, whether in battle or athletic competitions. She was a messenger (*angelos*) who sometimes used a trumpet to herald her message. As she flew, she brought the victor an insignia of victory – a crown, fillet,* palm, trophy of arms or naval trophy. Once back on earth, she took part in the libation or sacrifice made by the victor to thank the gods. When the Romans conquered the Greek world, they immediately embraced *Nike* as *Victoria*, a symbol of Rome's domination of the known world and an icon of the virtue of the Roman people.

***

Nike was the daughter of the Titan *Pallas* and the goddess *Styx*, and the sister of *Kratos* (Strength), *Bia* (Force) and *Zelos* (Zeal). *Pallas* was the Titan god of warcraft. During the Titanomachy,† *Pallas* fought against the Olympians – the new and powerful generation of gods led by *Zeus*. Unlike her husband *Pallas*, *Styx* chose the side of the Olympians during the Titanomachy. She even consigned her children – the goddesses *Kratos*, *Bia*, *Zelos* and *Nike* – to the services of *Zeus*. *Pallas* ended up dying at the hands of *Athena*, the daughter of *Zeus* and the goddess of wisdom and strategic warfare.

As a loyal battle companion of *Zeus*, *Nike* served him as his divine charioteer, circling the battlefield and bestowing praise, adulation and a laurel wreath to the victors. The laurel wreath remains not only a symbol of victory to this day but also signifies achievement; a person or organization awarded the Nobel Prize is a Nobel Laureate. *Zeus* was so pleased with the siblings that he ordered them to live with him in Olympos.

> At the time when Zeus entered upon the fight against the Titans, and called upon the gods for assistance, Nice and her two sisters were the first that came forward, and Zeus was so pleased with their readiness, that he caused them ever after to live with him in Olympus.[1]

---

* Ribbon or narrow strip of material used as a headband.
† A ten-year series of battles fought in Thessaly between the Titans fighting against the Olympians to decide which generation of gods would reign over the Universe; it ended in victory for the Olympians.

A ubiquitous national symbol of victory, *Nike* often stood by the sides of many ancient Greek statues of the Olympian gods and goddesses. She was also placed atop famous landmarks and monuments in ancient Greek cities as an *akroterion*.‡ Citizens believed that *Nike* could lead the city to victory against their foes. Moreover, the placing of statues or symbols of *Nike* in one's home was also common, considering that every individual had some sort of personal battle or problem that he or she had to go through in life. Having *Nike* on one's side, be it man or god, automatically conferred the person or god victory.

The Ancients knew that the patron goddess of victory had to be depicted in a manner that showed *all the ideal elements of battlefield victory – fitness, strength, agility, and youthfulness*. Because of this, *Nike* was often portrayed as a winged goddess. As the messenger of the Greek gods, she was shown in the finest clothes and ornaments, adorned with a gown of gold. *Nike* was sometimes pictured with the Staff of Hermes and golden winged sandals. It was said that the possession of the staff granted breathtaking speed and agility and allowed the holder to move between the land of the living and the land of the dead (*Hades*). Her wings allowed her to glide from one place to another, bringing victory to people that deserve it.

As victory, *Nike* was also considered an attribute as well as a goddess. In antiquity, the most celebrated representations of *Nike* were the 5th century BCE statues of *Athena* and *Zeus* which stood, respectively, within the Parthenon of Athens and the Temple of Zeus at Olympia. Her name was attached to the gods Zeus and Athena, for example, as *Athena Nike*, the deity of victory. Pausanias described the statue thusly:

> The statue of Athena is upright, with a tunic reaching to the feet, and on her breast the head of Medusa is worked in ivory. She holds a statue of Victory (*Nike*) that is approximately four cubits§ high.[2]

The gods – literally and figuratively – held victory in their hands. *Nike* was always closely associated with *Athena*, and in the case

---

‡ An architectural ornament placed on a flat pedestal and mounted at the apex or corner of the pediment (gable) of a building.
§ Approximately equal to the length of a forearm, 18 inches.

of *Zeus* and the pan-Hellenic games of Olympia, significant in her role as bestower of prizes. The statue of *Zeus* was considered one of the Seven Wonders of the Ancient World. Neither statue survives.

Interestingly, the temple of *Nike* bore a wingless *Nike* in service to *Athena*; this statue stood in the *cella*, or *naos*.** Although more often portrayed as a "winged victory" goddess, the *Athena Nike* statue's absence of wings led Athenians in later centuries to call it *Apteros Nike* or wingless victory. As time went on, the story evolved that the statue was deprived of wings so that it could never leave the city, thus ensuring enduring victory.

In keeping with her close association with battle in a warring society, *Nike* was also, on a few occasions, described as an attendant, minister and even daughter of *Ares* by Homer:

> Ares, exceeding in strength, chariot-rider, golden-helmed, doughty†† in heart, shield-bearer, Saviour of cities, harnessed in bronze, strong of arm, unwearying, mighty with the spear, O defence of Olympus, father of warlike Victory.[3]

***

Nike's attributes developed over time. While earlier descriptions during and shortly after her role in the Titanomachy emphasized her participation in the heat of battle, with time she became more aligned with the strategic wisdom of *Athena*.

As described in a speech attributed to the orator Lycurgus of Athens (c. 390–324 BCE):

> Alternatively [she stands] allegorically for the notion that *even winning is completely dependent on thought*; for thought contributes to victory, but being thoughtless and impetuous while fighting leads to defeat. When she has wings she symbolizes that aspect of the mind that is sharp and, so to speak, swift-winged; but when she is depicted without wings she represents that aspect of it that is peaceful and quiet and civil, that by which the things of the earth flourish, a boon

---

** The *cella* was the inner area of an ancient temple, especially one housing a hidden cult image in a Greek or Roman temple. Sometimes used interchangeably with *naos*, which was the temple or shrine itself.

†† Brave and persistent.

VICTORY AND RETREAT: *NIKE* AND *PALIOXIS* 221

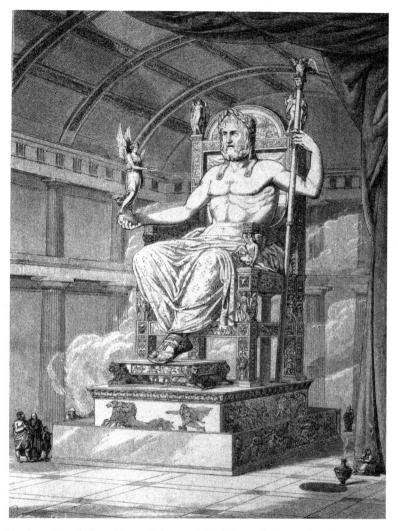

Jupiter (Zeus) sits with a miniature *Nike* (Victory) in one hand. Inspired by Greek statue of Zeus at Olympia by Pheidias, c. 1 CE.

of which the pomegranate in her right hand is a representation. Just as the helmet in her left [is a representation] of battle. Thus she has the same capability as Athena.[4]

Understandably, there was little room for defeat in Ancient Greek war culture, art, or literature. Battles would portray victory and defeat, to be sure, but attention was devoted to the victors.

The *Machae* or *Machai* were the spirits of battle and combat and were sons or daughters of *Eris*:

> But abhorred *Strife* bore ... *Fightings* also, *Battles*, *Murders*, *Manslaughters*, *Quarrels*, *Lying Words*, *Disputes*, *Lawlessness* and *Ruin*, all of one nature, and *Oath* who most troubles men upon earth when anyone willfully swears a false oath.[5]

The daemons *Homados* (Battle-Noise), *Alala* (War-Cry), *Proioxis* (Onrush), *Palioxis* (Backrush) and *Kydoimos* (Confusion) were closely associated with the *Machai*. They were accompanied in battlefields by other deities and spirits associated with war and death. *Palioxis* was the personification of backrush, flight and retreat in battle (as opposed to *Proioxis*). She is mentioned together with other personifications having to do with war. Among a show of force, backrush was eclipsed.

***

We often say we will defeat disease, conquer cancer, be victorious over ... the COVID-19 pandemic, or some other medical challenge. The metaphors doing battle with disease have long been a part of the portrayal of health care as curative and successful. And by any metric, it is a laudable goal.

However, "Across the world death is still viewed as a failure."[6] Health care professionals are trained to save people, not to let them die. From the little published literature that exists, refusal to admit failure drives physician reluctance more than anything else.[7] Doctors don't like to talk about death. It sounds too much like failure.[8] There may be relatively little difference in the psychology of the health care system facing defeat and failure from the psychology of the Ancients millennia ago.

Why have doctors been so bad at admitting defeat, and is there any evidence for believing that this might be going through an evolutionary change, even as we make medical advances at an unprecedented rate? Ironically, junior physicians and medical students currently may have a more balanced and sensitive view at the death bed than their elders because of a vastly different level of participation on the part of patients and families as well as the ecumenical availability of information about alternatives and the right to choose. Regardless of senior clinicians having achieved eminence, the difficulty and reluctance to admit helplessness and defeat often prevails, and may result in treating patients "to death."[9]

A recent legislative advance that enhances and even emboldens this discussion with patients is Medical Orders for Life-Sustaining Treatment (MOLST). A MOLST is a form that contains directions about CPR and other life-sustaining treatments (which anesthesiologists are often involved with) specific to a patient's current condition. Because it is a medical order, it must be signed and dated by a licensed state medical provider. This is different than an Advance Directive, which can contain a living will, organ donation requests, plans to donate one's body to science and the appointment of an agent to make health decisions if one becomes unconscious. For the MOLST statute to achieve its goal, physicians must be willing to *discuss* end of life decisions with their patients. In doing so, they must admit to their patients and to themselves that they may not be able to save their patients' lives.

Defeat at the end of life is a small part of the many defeats throughout one's professional life. For anyone in medicine for any length of time, mistakes, setbacks and failures will happen:

- An attempted central line caused a pneumothorax, or punctured a carotid artery
- An attempted tracheal intubation succeeded in intubating the esophagus.
- An attempt to treat low blood pressure with large amounts of intravenous fluid when the actual problem was heart failure; the extra fluid load only made the heart failure worse.

We have all had these "failures" in some form or another. It is how we overcome the failure that will make us succeed in medicine. We can learn from our mistakes. Even if no mistake was made, we can learn from our defeats.

An enlightened approach consists of several steps that have become more acknowledged in recent years. The first step is accepting the failure. It will hurt a little – and sometimes a lot. We may distract ourselves with something else, perhaps a rationalization or marginally plausible explanation, but that is a mistake and will not help in the long run. The second step is thinking deeply and critically about what could have been done differently. Was this preventable? or predictable? Were you in a hurry? Did you have all your equipment ready? Did you have a Plan B? While many of these questions are typically asked at a Morbidity and Mortality meeting, a staple of most department's conferences reviewing adverse outcomes, only you know what you were thinking and feeling at the time these events occurred. Only you get to re-live in your mind's eye your experience; everyone else is just guessing. The third step is to reframe the criticism, create new rules and turn them into a developmental/educational mindset, with a belief that failure is integral to professional development and provides a compass for future growth. On the emotional side, the fourth step is to create a multi-pillar support system, personally and professionally. The personal support system will consist of family and friends who will understand your strengths and especially your vulnerabilities. The professional support system can be on an informal level, but that does not work as well as a more formal system scheduling a recurring meeting so that it becomes support-over-time. Because of entropy, this always has a tendency to fall apart much more readily than the personal support network. The last step is to progress beyond the failure or defeat. Not to forget but to harvest wisdom in order to be better (more victorious) in the future and also enhance your ability to teach that to others – an act of kindness – *philophrosyne.*

Another advancing concept in professional growth and development is the idea of professional coaching in medicine. It operationalizes a concept in numerous other domains that is not generally practiced in medicine:

> in our traditional educational and professional process there is a perception that after a defined amount of time a student no longer needs instruction. It is presumed that after a certain point you go the rest of the way on your own by practicing what you have learned.[10]

This editorial extract was written in response to a thoughtful essay by Dr. Atul Gawande in the *New Yorker* in 2011 when he concluded "Coaching done well may be the most effective intervention designed for human performance." This followed his beneficial experience, as a surgeon well into practice, being coached by an admired prior mentor.[11] This is distinctly different from simulation training in medicine, developed over the last 30 years.

***

How does removal from the context of war change *Nike?* Can there be no victory without war? For the Ancients, that may very well have been the case, although much of life was seen as a contest and Victory was important in sports as well as oration. Is health care a contest in contemporary society? In the minds of many the answer is yes.

Doctors are not gods, and do not hold victory in their hands like *Zeus* and *Athena*. But if the focus of victory is enlarged *beyond* the defeat of the disease affecting the patient and incorporated into the growth in wisdom and influence impact in the larger context of society and the practitioner, it will be worthy of Nike, goddess of victory and her reward to the victorious – *laurel nobilis*.

References

1. Hesiod. *The Homeric Hymns and Homerica. Theogony*. Cambridge, MA, Harvard University Press, 1914, line 382, ff.
2. Pausanias. *Description of Greece*. Cambridge, MA, Harvard University Press, 1918, Jones WHS, Ormerod, HA trans. 1.24.7.
3. Homer. *The Homeric Hymns and Homerica*. Homeric Hymns, Cambridge, MA, Harvard University Press, 1914.
4. Suidas. *Nike Athena, Byzantine Greek Lexicon, C 10th CE*. www.cs.uky.edu/~raphael/sol/sol-entries/nu/384 Accessed 4/21/21.
5. Hesiod. *The Homeric Hymns and Homerica. Theogony*. Cambridge, MA, Harvard University Press, 1914, line 226.
6. Daud M, Lee Chee C, Taib F. Medical students' preparedness as junior doctors on palliative care issues: a single centre study. *Education in Medicine Journal* 2016; 8: 3–14.
7. Brown A, Miles T. Refusing to admit defeat: physicians' reluctance to discuss end of life care. *Palliat Med Care* 2016; 3: 1–2.
8. Brown S. Why many doctors still find it difficult to talk about dying with patients. *CMAJ* 2019; 191: e22–3.

9. Gould D. Forum: never say die – why are doctors so reluctant to admit defeat? *New Scientist* 1990.
10. Byyny R. Mentoring and coaching in medicine (editorial), *The Pharos, Alpha Omega Alpha* 2012: 1–3.
11. Gawande A. The coach in the operating room. *The New Yorker* 2011: 16.

Part VII

SOCIETY

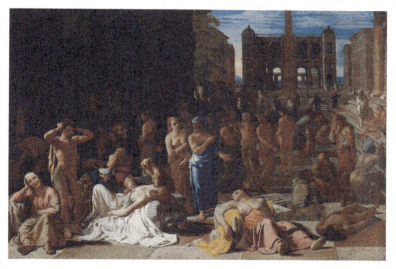

The Plague of Athens, c. 1652–1654. Michiel Sweerts (1618–1664) (Michiel Sweerts, public domain, via Wikimedia Commons.)

The Plague of Athens was an epidemic that devastated that city-state during the second year of the Peloponnesian War (430 BCE). It is believed to have entered Athens through *Piraeus*, the city's port and sole source of food and supplies. The plague returned twice, in 429 BCE and in the winter of 427/426 BCE. Some 30 pathogens have been suggested as the cause. Currently the leading theory is moldy food containing immunosuppressive mycotoxins produced by certain *Fusarium* microfungi. Scarcity of food may have forced the population of overcrowded Athens to consume any food, even when moldy.

Toxigenic fungi and mycotoxins have been identified as remotely as 10,000 years ago when mankind first began to cultivate crops and store them from one season to the next. The historian Thucydides, who contracted the disease himself and survived, described the epidemic and its effect on physicians:

> Not many days after their arrival in Attica the plague first began to show itself among the Athenians. It was said that it had broken out in many places previously in the neighborhood of Lemnos and elsewhere; but a pestilence of such extent and mortality was nowhere remembered. Neither were the physicians at first of any service, ignorant as they were of the proper way to treat it, but they died themselves the most thickly, as they visited the sick most often; nor did any human art succeed any better. Supplications in the temples, divinations, and so forth were found equally futile, till the overwhelming nature of the disaster at last put a stop to them altogether.[1]

In overcrowded Athens, the disease killed an estimated 25 percent of the population.

When Aristotle stated that "Man is a political animal",[2] what he meant was that man is an animal who lives in a *polis*. The *polis* was a "face-to-face" community – a community that was sufficiently small that people would have known, or at least recognized, a significant percentage of the entire community. As a result, the social and political structures of your *polis* would have bound you very closely to your fellow citizens and to your peers. This meant, for instance, that you took slavery for granted and had an intense suspicion and dislike of non-Greeks. In many cases, you would have an intense, visceral dislike of Greeks who weren't from your *polis*. And, finally, you led a life that was much more like the lives of all your fellow citizens, simply because there were far fewer life-choices available.

Although *poleis* were each a unique cultural and political unit, the common features of culture, language and religion also meant that there were feelings of connection between *poleis*.

Like-minded *poleis* often made political alliances for mutual protection. A Pan-Hellenic attitude between *poleis* was manifested in two specific circumstances – wars against non-Greek enemies (e.g., the Persian Wars of the 5th century BCE) and Pan-Hellenic festivals such as the Olympic Games held at Olympia every four years.

The development of rational (non-supernatural) medicine on the islands of Kos and Knidos in western Asia Minor provided an intriguing multicultural contrast to the *poleis*. Early Greek medicine inherited knowledge from many older sources and cultivated broad connections with other lands and cultures. Due to their geographical location, the Greeks were exposed to the influence of Egyptian, Assyro-Babylonian, Mesopotamian, Phoenician and Minoan civilizations. In addition, they also learned a great amount from lay and ancient Jewish medicine, especially with regard to sanitary laws, prevention and prophylaxis.

In the late 4th century BCE, Alexander the Great and his successors spread the idea of the *polis* throughout the Macedonian empire, typically with resettled Greeks acting as the ruling elite and the local population becoming subject farmers. *Poleis*, therefore, became less significant in terms of independent political power but continued to be significant as sources of civic pride.

References

1. Thucydides. *The Peloponnesian War*. London, J. M. Dent, 1910, 2.47.
2. Aristotle. *Politics*. Vol. 21 *Aristotle in 23 Volumes*. Cambridge, MA, Harvard University Press, 1944. 1.1253a.

23
LAW AND ORDER/LAWLESSNESS, DISORDER AND RUIN: *NOMOS* AND *EUNOMIA/DYSNOMIA* AND *ATE*

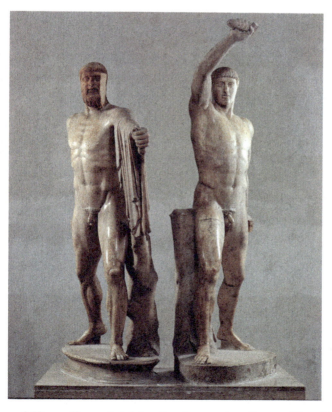

Statue of *Harmodius* and *Aristogeiton*, known together as *Tiranicidas*, Roman copy of the Athenian version by Kritios and Nesiotes.

After the establishment of Athenian democracy, *Kleisthenes*[*] (c. 570 – c. 508 BCE) commissioned a statue of *Harmodius* and *Aristogeiton*, together known as *Tyrranicides* ("killers of a tyrant"). It was the first commission of its kind, and the very first statue to be paid for out of public funds, as the two were the first Greeks *considered by their countrymen* worthy of having statues raised to them. Notwithstanding their executions for the murder of the tyrant Hipparchus at the hands of his brother Hippias, they were remembered by the poet Simonides (c. 556–468 BCE) with "A marvelous great light shone upon Athens when Aristogeiton and Harmodios slew Hipparchus."[1]

They were punished by law; they were immortalized by justice.

***

Nomos

Nomos was the personified spirit of law and was the husband of *Eusebeia* (Piety) and the father of *Dike* (Justice). He was considered an aspect of *Zeus* rather than a separate divinity. According to Pindar:

> The holy king of Gods and men I call, celestial Law [Nomos], the righteous seal of all;
> The seal which stamps whate'er the earth contains, Nature's firm basis, and the liquid plains:
> Stable, and starry, of harmonious frame, preserving laws eternally the same:
> Thy all-composing pow'r in heaven appears, connects its frame, and props the starry spheres;
> And shakes weak Envy with tremendous sound, toss'd by thy arm in giddy whirls around.
> 'Tis thine, the life of mortals to defend, and crown existence with a blessed end;
> For thy command and alone, of all that lives order and rule to ev'ry dwelling gives:
> Ever observant of the upright mind, and of just actions the companion kind;

---

[*] An ancient Athenian lawgiver credited with reforming the constitution of Athens and setting it on a democratic footing in 508 BCE as well as increasing the power of the citizens' assembly therefore reducing the power of the nobility over Athenian politics.

Foe to the lawless, with avenging ire, their steps involving in destruction dire.
Come, bless, abundant pow'r, whom all revere, by all desir'd, with favr'ing mind draw near;
Give me thro' life, on thee to fix my fight, and ne'er forsake the equal paths of right.[2]

Eusebeia, the wife of *Nomos* (from *eu-* meaning "well" and *sebas* meaning "reverence") personified behavior appropriate to the gods. The root *seb-* meant sacred awe and reverence and was associated with danger and flight. The sense of reverence originally described was fear of the gods as motivation for lawful behavior. In Classical Greece it meant behaving as tradition dictates in one's social relationships and towards the gods. One demonstrates *eusebeia* to the gods by performing the customary acts of respect (festivals, prayers, sacrifices, public devotions). By extension, one honors the gods by showing proper respect to elders, masters, rulers and everything under the protection of the gods. The Roman equivalent was *Pietas*.

Asebeia was the opposite of *Eusebeia*, and was considered a crime in Athens, punishable by death or exile. *Dyssebeia* was also considered a crime.

Law and Nature: *Nomos and Physis*[3]

Nomos represented the unwritten customs as well as the written laws of a society. In large part due to the travels required by war, a heightened awareness of how *nomōi* differed between cultures and over time became part of Greek society's corpus, amplifying societal insecurities about preserving their values and surviving. *Physis*, or nature, is agreed-upon reality through direct observation and is the basis for the word "physics," the study of matter, motion, energy and force. *Physis* also involved natural growth to a mature state, in order to flourish.

In the 5th and 4th centuries BCE, playwrights, orators and historians as well as philosophers entered the vigorous debate of *nomos* vs. *physis* in the *polis*. One of the themes of Sophocles' Antigone was that the laws of the state may conflict with natural law (*nomima*) of the gods. That this was an active and public subject was reflected in Sophocles' play Antigone. Antigone buried her brother, Polynices, in defiance of the edict of King Creon, who represented the rule of the state. Antigone defended her action by claiming divine sanction (the same justification as Creon's), but in accordance with the law, she was buried (alive) and died, although not by asphyxiation ... she hanged herself. Creon's son, who was in love with Antigone, died by suicide and his mother the Queen also killed herself in despair over her son's death. Antigone reached out from the grave and destroyed her adversary, Creon.

This plot line highlighted the contrast between the *nomōi* of a state and the *physis* of nature.

The Greek orator *Antiphon* of Rhamnus (480–411 BCE) argued that laws are generally antithetical to nature, and that the individual's interests will be best served by following nature when legal punishment can be avoided. He proposed that justice (with a small "j") consists of not breaking the laws and customs of the state in which you are a citizen, yet he also acknowledged "nature" might be antithetical to social harmony.

Other champions of *physis* suggested that as a law of nature, the naturally superior should seize political control and should freely indulge their desires. Thucydides' (c. 460–400 BCE) Melian Dialogue was one example. During the Peloponnesian War in the 5th century BCE, Athens demanded that the small island of Melos, an ally of Sparta, surrender. The Melians thought this both unjust and unwise – why not simply allow Melos to remain neutral? Unmoved, the Athenians conquered the island, and "put to death all the grown men whom they took, and sold the women and children for slaves, and subsequently sent out five hundred colonists and inhabited the place themselves."[4]

Might Makes Right: Wasn't That *Physis* as Well?

Traditionally *physis* had been employed by aristocrats to support the notion of a superior class naturally fitted to rule, but by the late 5th century BCE appeals to *physis* were also being used to refute this claim and question the social hierarchy. *Antiphon*, for example, claimed that there was no natural distinction between the high- and low-born, or between Greek and non-Greek. He continued this antithesis against slavery, racial discrimination and class struggle. Contrast this with Plato's recounting of a dialogue between Crito and Socrates (Crito, 51d) when Socrates argues that each citizen, by freely electing to remain in their city and receiving the benefits of its protection, has made an implicit contract to abide by its *nomōi*. Both Plato and Aristotle sought to resolve the nomos/physis antithesis by claiming that the creation of *nomōi* is an essential part of human *physis*.

Eunomia

Eunomia was the goddess of good order and lawful conduct. In the *polis* (i.e., "politically") she was associated with the internal stability of a state, including the enactment of good laws and the maintenance of civil order. As one of the *Horai*, goddesses of the seasons, she was also the spring-time goddess of green pastures. Her sisters were the goddesses *Dike* (Justice) and *Eirene* (Peace), daughters of Divine Law according to Hesiod:

> Next he [Zeus] led away bright *Themis* (Divine Law) who bare the *Horai* (Horae, Seasons), and *Eunomia* (Good Order), *Dike* (Justice), and blooming *Eirene* (Irene, Peace), who mind the works of mortal men.[5]

Pindar renders a more trenchant description of the role of law and order in protecting the wealthy and ensuring the status quo:

> I shall recognize prosperous Corinth, the portal of Isthmian Poseidon, glorious in her young men. There dwell *Eunomia* and her sisters, the secure foundation of cities: *Dike*, and *Eirene*, who was raised together with her, the guardians of wealth for men, the golden daughters of wise *Themis*. They are resolute in repelling *Hybris*, the bold-tongued mother of *Koros*.[6]

Dysnomia and Ate

Dysnomia ("lawlessness"), the opposite of *Eunomia*, was imagined by Hesiod among the daughters of "abhorred Eris" ("Strife") as the spirit of lawlessness and poor civil order. She was a companion of *Adikia* (Injustice), *Ate* (Ruin) and *Hybris* (Violence). According to Hesiod:

But abhorred *Eris* (Strife) bare painful *Ponos* (Toil), and *Lethe* (Forgetfulness), and *Limos* (Starvation), and the *Algea* (Pains), full of weeping, the *Hysminai* (Fightings) and the *Makhai* (Battles), the *Phonoi* (Murders) and the *Androktasiai* (Manslaughters), the *Neikea* (Quarrels), the *Pseudo-Logoi* (Lies), the *Amphilogiai* (Disputes), and *Dysnomia* (Lawlessness) and *Ate* (Ruin), who share one another's natures, and *Horkos* (Oath).[7]

Solon (c. 630–560 BCE), an Athenian statesman whose criticisms of the Athenian political system failed in the short term but ultimately contributed to Athenian democracy, offered:

> This is what my heart bids me teach the Athenians, that *Dysnomia* (Lawlessness) brings the city countless ills, but *Eunomia* (Lawfulness) reveals all that is orderly and fitting, and often places fetters[†] round the unjust. She makes the rough smooth, puts a stop to excess, weakens insolence (*hubris*), dries up the blooming of ruin (*ate*), straightens out crooked judgements, tames deeds of pride, and puts an end to acts of sedition and to the anger of grievous strife.[8]

Atë was the Greek goddess of mischief, delusion, ruin, and folly. As a verb, *Atë* also refers to an action performed by a hero that leads to their death or downfall. Her power was countered by the *Litai* (Prayers) which followed in her wake.

However, Homer paints a pessimistic picture in the Iliad of the efficacy of prayer over ruin:

> even the very gods can bend ... Their hearts by incense and reverent vows and libations and the savour of sacrifice do men turn from wrath with supplication, whenso any man transgresseth and doeth sin. For Prayers are the daughters of great Zeus, halting and wrinkled and of eyes askance, and they are ever mindful to follow in the steps of Sin. Howbeit Sin is strong and fleet of foot, wherefore she far out-runneth them all, and goeth before them over the face of all the earth

---

† A chain or manacle used to restrain a prisoner, typically placed around the ankles.

making men to fall, and Prayers follow after, seeking to heal the hurt.[9]

Ate shared the same numerous siblings as *Dysnomia*, all born from *Eris* (Strife).

***

Plato's *Republic* is concerned with the nature of justice and how it operates in a social context. Socrates declared that justice is the quality of the well-ordered soul that results in each person "practic[ing] one of the functions in the city, that one for which [he is] naturally most fit." Justice is each person minding his or her own business. By defining justice in this way, Socrates conveys that each individual fits a specific role in society, and that social harmony is at its peak when each individual works in that role.[10]

The customary "laws" of medicine that have educated, trained and provided cultural guidelines have traditionally kept physicians within their "lane" as clinicians, scientists and educators. Although that parochial view is rapidly changing across medical school and practice curricula, it is worthwhile thinking about the forces that contributed (and continue to contribute, although in dwindling numbers with generational changes) to the rabid individualism of medical practice.

The Flexner report of 1910 and its source of funding, the Carnegie Foundation, gave rise to our current system of medical education.[11] It remains characterized by competitive admission criteria, traditional teaching models and the scientific method. Although optimal comprehensive patient care has always included assessments of the patient's environment and family factors, social, societal and environmental influences did not appear in the curriculum but rather were cultivated in the office, through face-to-face community interactions or through house call visits. Such non-medical assessments were not part of the *nomos* of medical education.

In 2019, more than 100 years after the Flexner Report, Goldfarb ignited a reactionary tempest when he cast doubt on the evolving values of incorporating social justice into traditional aspects of the medical training curriculum.[12] In a *Wall Street Journal* Opinion essay, he accused the American College of Physicians of "stepping out of its lane" after issuing statements about gun control – as a public health issue. Swift and in most cases harsh responses followed, including those from his (former) medical school about societal influences on who gets sick, who gets care, and where, and how.

Yet Goldfarb is not alone in his opinion. He desires a return to a *status quo ante* that is no longer natural. The natural law of medicine, staying in one's own professional lane, is no longer natural.

Rather, collaborative learning and clinical practice have been increasingly recognized as natural. The freedom of the rugged individual as a medical sensibility has developed into a recognition of medical practice as a collective responsibility, whether it is the operating room team on a microscopic level, or the effort to develop a COVID-19 vaccine on a worldwide level.

Current national and international crises call for careful analysis, understanding, policy creation and intervention. Not uncommonly, medical intervention and acute and critical care will be part of the response. Advocacy – promoting the role of science and evidenced-based medicine in the creation of health and social policy – has been treated as if it's unscientific and therefore a lesser endeavor, even though, through their various professional organizations' public policy positions, most physicians think it's just the opposite.[13] Voices of health care workers including physicians can provide facts and data as well as context and meaning, underscoring the importance of Voice. Beyond *Paregoros*, this would also be the goal of *Kalliope* (see Chapters 19 and 20).

Nomos has relegated a large percentage of time spent with patients to box checking over actual patient care, the kind of care that patients care about. An imbalance of *nomos* and *physis* – medicine's undervaluing of the power of talk – has implications far beyond documentation of an "encounter."[14]

***

Law and Order are not the same; laws support social order and may be unaligned with natural order. The obvious changes in knowledge, science, and clinical practice and the evolving natural order of understanding the contributions of societal tensions, climate change and political regime-ism demand that a much broader view be incorporated and integrated into our care of patients and how we comport ourselves as a profession.

References

1. Edmonds J. *Lyra Graeca: Being the Remains of All the Greek Lyric Poets from Eumelus to Timotheus excepting Pindar.* Vol. 2. London and New York, William Heinemann & G. P. Putnam's Sons, 1931.
2. The Orphic Hymns. *The Hymns of Orpheus.* Philadelphia, PA, University of Pennsylvania Press, 1999.
3. Hobbs A. *Physis and Nomos, Routledge Encyclopedia of Philosophy.* Milton, Taylor & Francis, 1998.
4. Thucydides. *The History of the Peloponnesian War,* Vol. 17. Sixteenth Year of the War. The Melian Conference – Fate of Melos. www.mtholyoke.edu/acad/intrel/melian.htm Accessed 4/21/21.
5. Hesiod. *The Homeric Hymns and Homerica, Theogony.* Cambridge, MA, Harvard University Press, 1914, line 901 ff.
6. Pindar. *Olympian 13 For Xenophon of Corinth Foot Race and Pentathlon 464 B.C., Svarlien, DA trans. Perseus Project.* Medford, MA, Tufts University, 1990.
7. Hesiod. *The Homeric Hymns and Homerica, Theogony.* Cambridge, MA, Harvard University Press, 1914, p 230 ff.
8. Gerber D. *Greek Elegiac Poetry From the Seventh to the Fifth Centuries BC. Loeb Classical Library.* Vol. 258 Cambridge, MA, Harvard University Press, 1999.
9. Homer. *The Iliad.* Cambridge, MA, Harvard University Press, 1924, p 498 ff.
10. Plato. *Republic Plato in Twelve Volumes.* Cambridge, MA, Harvard University Press, 1969. Plat. Rep. 4. 433a ff.
11. Bleakley A. *Embracing the Collective Through Medical Education, Advances in Health Sciences Education, 10/30/2020 edition,* Springer.
12. Goldfarb S. *Take Two Aspirin and Call Me by my Pronouns, Wall Street Journal.* 9/12/2019. New York, New York Times Corporation, 2019.
13. Fleck L. *Health Care and Social Justice: Just Take Two Aspirin for Your Tumor If You Cannot Afford Your Cancer Care, MSU Bioethics.* Michigan, Center for Bioethics and Social Justice: Bioethics in the News: Michigan State University, 2019.
14. Rosenbaum L. No Cure without Care – Soothing Science Skepticism. *New Engl J Med* 2021; 384: 1462–1465.

24
JUSTICE AND DEMOCRACY: *DIKE* AND *DEMOKRATIA*

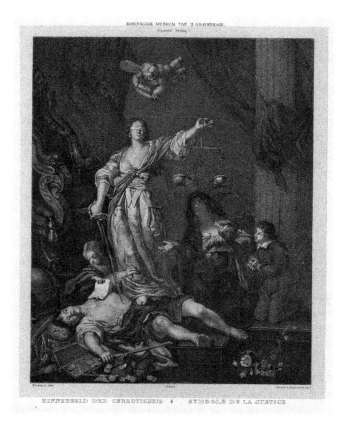

The Triumph of Justice (*Justitia* (L); *Dike* (Gr)), c. 1828. (after Gabriel Metsu (1629–1667)). Justice is standing at the center, blindfolded and holding scales while pointing her sword at a man who lies on his back in left foreground, coins scattered around him and a disguising mask positioned next to his face. (British Museum, public domain, via Wikimedia Commons.)

DOI: 10.1201/9781003201328-32

Law and justice have an intriguing relationship, which should be very close but is often very far apart. Law, like pregnancy is a binary concept – you are or aren't (lawful or pregnant). Justice is not as simple, and its application is even more complex.

***

Dike was the goddess of justice and the spirit of moral order and fair judgement. According to Hesiod, she was fathered by *Zeus* with his second consort, *Themis*. *Dike* and *Themis* were both personifications of justice. While *Themis* was the goddess of divine law, *Dike* was the goddess of the law of man. She was depicted as a young woman carrying a balance scale and wearing a laurel wreath while her Roman counterpart (*Justitia*) was outfitted similarly but also blind-folded.

Her opposite was *Adikia*, the personified spirit of injustice and wrongdoing. She was depicted as an ugly, barbarian woman with tattooed skin. Pausanias unambiguously described the intense harshness of their relationship as shown on the Chest of Kypselos:

> A beautiful woman is punishing an ugly one, choking her with one hand and with the other striking her with a staff. It is Justice who thus treats Injustice.[1]

Themis also represented the law and undisputed order. She created divine laws that governed everything including the Olympian gods. While *Themis* was goddess of divine justice, morality amongst the gods. *Dike* was to rule over human justice. In her theogony, *Themis* had three supporting sets of offspring: the *Horai* (*Eunomia* [fair order], *Dike* [trial] and *Eirene* [peace]), the *Moirai* (the Fates, or destiny) and the *Nymphs* (Prophecy), as well as the virgin *Astraea*. With the progression toward the Athenian democracy of the 4th century BCE this theogony was replaced by *dikaiosynē*,* Plato's cardinal virtue, justice.

The special importance of Justice to mankind was acknowledged by Hesiod's description of Divine benevolence:

---

* Adding "syne" to the end of an adjective turns that adjective into an abstract noun, so dikai (justice) + *syne* = dikaisyne (a state of justice, or "fairness").

For the son of Cronos has ordained this law for men, that fishes and beasts and winged fowls should devour one another ..."[2]

However, Justice was not a pushover, hence the sword along with the scales in the above illustration as well as her contentious relationship with *Adikia*. *Dike* sat beside her father, *Zeus*, weighing justice and meting out harsh judgement:

And there is virgin Justice, the daughter of Zeus, who is honored and reverenced among the gods who dwell on Olympus, and whenever anyone hurts her with lying slander, she sits beside her father, Zeus the son of Cronos, and tells him of men's wicked heart, until the people pay for the mad folly of their princes.[2]

Dike's name, Δικη, in Ancient Greek meant behavior in accordance with nature, without a moral connotation. It was only later, as noted, that the name came to be more closely identified with "justice."

This shift was an evolutionary process. The 6th-century BCE lawgiver Solon (c. 630–560 BCE) promoted *dike* – law-abiding conduct – as part of a general program of *eunomia* (good, civil law and order) in the *polis*. He also spoke of his legislation as providing a straight *dike* (judicial process) for every Athenian citizen. For the 5th-century philosopher Heraklitus (c. 500 BCE), *dike* was a cosmic force of order and balance, which was in keeping with his theories of universal flux or constant change and balance of opposites. He therefore concluded that *dike* is *eris* (strife) (see Chapter 11, *Eris* and *Harmonia*). Popularized to the public by tragedian playwrights of the time, *dike* was portrayed as a cosmic force in the sense of punishment or retribution, which certainly served the law-and-order goals of the *polis*. Plato's Protagoras relates to his Dialogue partner Socrates the story of how the gods gave *dike*, together with *aidōs* (respect) to *all humans*. He concluded from this that *dike* was *necessary* for the survival of human society.[3]

Throughout this time, *dike* in all its meanings – as goddess, cosmic force and even judicial process – remained something external to mankind. In the 4th century BCE, Plato transitioned justice to a personal virtue of individuals, and that's when *dike* became *dikaiosynē*. The Sophist *Thrasymachus* (c. 459 – c. 400 BCE), however, held that justice was the invention of those in power and called obedience to these laws "justice."

Demosthenes (384–322 BCE), who orated (in defense) of *Aristogeiton* (see Chapter 23) sternly warned jurors, reminding them of their fealty to the *polis* and *eunomia* as well as Divine Justice:

> You must magnify the Goddess of Order who loves what is right and preserves every city and every land; and before you cast your votes, each juryman must reflect that he is being watched by hallowed and inexorable Justice, who, as Orpheus, that prophet of our most sacred mysteries, tells us, sits beside the throne of Zeus and oversees all the works of men. Each must keep watch and ward lest he shame that goddess, from whom everyone that is chosen by lot derives his name of juror, because he has this day received a sacred trust from the laws, from the constitution, from the fatherland, – the duty of guarding all that is fair and right and beneficial in our city.[4]

***

The basis of justice, for many people, refers to fairness, but there are a number of recognized contexts. *Social justice* is the notion that everyone deserves equal economic, political, and social opportunities regardless of race, gender, or religion. *Distributive justice* refers to the equitable allocation of assets in society. *Environmental justice* is the fair treatment of all people with regard to environmental burdens and benefits. *Restorative or corrective justice* seeks to make whole those who have suffered unfairly. *Retributive justice* seeks to punish wrongdoers objectively and proportionately. And *procedural justice* refers to implementing legal decisions in accordance with fair and unbiased processes. Legal and political systems that maintain law and order are desirable, but they cannot sustain either unless they also achieve justice.

Social justice is increasingly recognized as an integral part of medical education, training and practice, albeit not without some controversy (see Chapter 23). Frankly, it is hard to achieve because its attainment requires a high degree of selflessness – and most of us are selfish. Human nature is such that we tend to prate about social justice if our individual interests are not threatened; genuine social justice indeed threatens very many people's individual interests.

As the Ancients feared, in the effort toward justice, modifications of extant forces in social justice can easily upset the social order. As was true in Ancient Greece, human society today continues to be stratified; the system tends to protect itself best that way. Pursuit of social justice would require that structure to be critically examined and reconstructed or dismantled, and everybody brought to the same level. This prospect is terrifying to many people, including the powerful who control the society. So it was in the *polis*, and so it continues today.

Finally, social justice has relatively few champions. Those who are in higher statuses have learned to enjoy them; those in lower statuses have learned to endure them. Everyone seems to "know their place," a repeat of Plato's quote from Crito. By defining justice in this way, Plato (as Socrates) means that each individual fits a specific role in society, and that social harmony is at its peak when each individual works in that role.[5]

***

Democracy (Greek; from *demos* "people" and *kratos* "rule") is a form of government in which the people have the authority to choose their governing legislators. In our contemporary understanding, its foundations include freedom of assembly and speech, inclusiveness and equality, membership, consent, voting, right to life and minority rights.

The term appeared in the 5th century BCE to denote the political systems then existing in Greek city-states, notably Athens, to mean "rule of the people," in contrast to aristocracy (*aristokratía*), meaning "rule of an elite." The political system of Classical Athens, for example, granted democratic citizenship to free men and excluded slaves and women from political participation. Athenian democracy was a direct democracy with two distinguishing features: the random selection of ordinary citizens to fill the few existing government administrative and judicial offices and a legislative assembly consisting of all Athenian citizens. While all eligible citizens were allowed to speak and vote in the assembly, Athenian citizenship excluded women, slaves, foreigners and men under 20 years of age; large parts of the Athenian populace, in some estimates 85 percent, were excluded from democracy. In virtually all democratic governments throughout ancient and modern history, democratic citizenship consisted of an elite class, until full enfranchisement was won for all adult citizens in most modern democracies through the suffrage movements of the 19th and 20th centuries.

A deeper look at the traditional etymology for democracy provides another interpretation. The two Greek words *demos*, meaning "the common people," and *kratos*, meaning "rule" may have drifted over millennia from their original meaning. For example, the word *demos* did not originally refer to "common people"; rather it referred to districts within Attica, the region that constituted the city-state of Athens. Each citizen of Attica, regardless of where he eventually resided (foreigners, women and slaves were all excluded from citizenship), was known by his *demos*. To participate in political affairs, each citizen had to be registered as a member of a *demos*. Thus *demos* eventually came to be associated with people from different regions of Attica. The original meaning of *demos* remains with us today in the English words *demographics* (which is not a homogenization of general human characteristics but rather characteristics related to a group of people living within the same region), *endemic* (which refers to characteristics that are unique to a particular region), *pandemic* (which refers to all regions and the people therein) and *academy*. The ancient Greeks, however, did have other words besides *demos* that either meant or related to the idea of "common people." One such word, *idiotes*, meant "unskilled person, private person, commoner, plebeian, layman" but eventually came to be a derogatory reference to people who did not participate in public life. It is, sadly, from *idiotes* that we get the English word idiot. Another ancient Greek word meaning "common people," "people of the nation" or "people assembled" was *laos*. It is from *laos* that we derive layman and laity.

Since *kratos* can be translated as "power," democracy has a literal root meaning of "the power of the people." Here again in contemporary interpretation, the power of the people is therefore the authority to decide matters by majority rule.[6]

However, careful examination according to historical context reveals that when it came to categorizing governance regimes, Greek names typically divide into terms with an *-arche* suffix or a *-kratos* suffix. *Aristokratia* (from *hoi aristoi*: the excellent), *isokratia* (from isos: equal) and *anarchia* are classical regime names that fall into the *-arche/-kratos* grouping. *Kratos*, when it is used as a regime-type suffix, becomes power in the sense of strength, enablement, or "capacity to do things."[6] *Demokratia*, which emerged as a regime-type with a *demos* in the setting of the Athenian Revolution refers to a *demos'* collective capacity to do things publicly – to make things happen. *Demokratia* is not just "the power of the demos" but rather "the empowered *demos*" – the *demos* gaining a collective capacity to effect public change. And it is not just a matter of control of a *polis* but also the collective strength and ability to act within that *polis*. This was the significance of the *demos'* collective strength first demonstrated during the Athenian Revolution of 508–507 BCE.

Demosthenes, in his oratory *Against Meidias*, exhorted jurors about the collective power they held in the enforcement of the words of the law:

> For if you would only examine and consider the question, what it is that gives you who serve on juries such power and authority in all state-affairs, whether the State empanels two hundred of you or a thousand or any other number, you would find that it is not that you alone of the citizens are drawn up under arms, not that your physical powers are at their best and strongest, not that you are in the earliest prime of manhood; it is due to no cause of that sort but simply to the strength of the laws.
>
> And what is the strength of the laws? If one of you is wronged and cries aloud, will the laws run up and be at his side to assist him? No; they are only written texts and incapable of such action. Wherein then resides their power? In yourselves, if only you support them and make them all-powerful to help him who needs them. So the laws are strong through you and you through the laws.
>
> Therefore you must help them as readily as any man would help himself if wronged; you must consider that you

share in the wrongs done to the laws, by whomsoever they are found to be committed; and no excuse—neither public services, nor pity, nor personal influence, nor forensic skill, nor anything else—must be devised whereby anyone who has transgressed the laws shall escape punishment.[7]

***

As a *demos*, physicians and all health professionals are part of a global community, especially today. Clinical ideas are shared, discoveries are made, and science is advanced with unprecedented speed through conferences, publications, the Internet, and lately, Zoom and other media platforms. There has never been a time when a global *demos* in medicine has existed with such immediacy.

This provides the context for an augmentation of medical professionalism, incorporating civic engagement and social justice activism as inherent to the current core role of physicians. This was poignantly expressed by a colleague and friend in a recent publication:

> I obtained an MPH at the Harvard School of Public Health in 2009 with a concentration in global health. At that time, the public health community viewed the idea of an anesthesiologist interested in public health, much less global health, as not only particularly strange, but it was also unclear if anesthesiologists even understood the nature of a true public health issue. I was told that TB, malaria, and HIV were real problems (which is true), while lack of access to safe and effective surgery and anesthesia was absolutely not a big problem (which is patently false). Surgery and anesthesia were viewed as health care interventions that were too expensive and technology driven to be implemented in low- and middle-income countries.[8]

This is *especially* important for nonprimary care specialists in surgery and anesthesiology,[9] who have remained, for the large part, "private" with regard to public health – until this year with the COVID-19 pandemic.

Civic advocacy is a neglected component of surgical and anesthesiology residency training, but it need no longer be as long as we can bring the *demos* of the surgical team together with the actionable *kratos* of their knowledge, skills and wisdom.

References

1. Pausanias. *Description of Greece.* Cambridge, MA, Harvard University Press, 1918. p 5.18.2.
2. Hesiod. *Works and Days. The Homeric Hymns and Homerica.* Cambridge, MA, Harvard University Press, 1914. pp 256–62; 275 ff.
3. Plato. *Protagoras. Plato in Twelve Volumes.* Cambridge, MA, Harvard University Press, 1967, l. 323a ff.
4. Demosthenes. *Against Aristogeiton (Oration).* Cambridge, MA, Harvard University Press, 1939, l. 25.11.
5. Plato. *Republic: Plato in Twelve Volumes.* Cambridge, MA, Harvard University Press, 1969. Plat. Rep. 4. 433a ff.
6. Ober J. *The Original Meaning of "Democracy": Capacity to Do Things, not majority rule.* Presented at: American Political Science Association Meetings. Philadelphia, PA, 2007.
7. Demosthenes. *Demosthenes: Against Meidias. Demosthenes.* Cambridge, MA, Harvard University Press, 1939, l. 223–5 ff.
8. McClain C, Stankey M. *Anessthesiology and Its Role in Functional Surgical Systems. ASA Monitor.* Chicago, IL, American Society of Anesthesiologists, 2021, pp 24–5.
9. Chawla K, Jayaram A, McClain C. The missing chapter: the education of surgery and anesthesiology trainees as civic advocates. *Ann Surg.* 2021; 273: e125–6.

POSTFACE

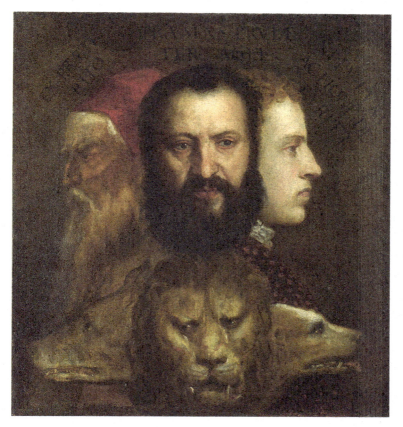

Titian's (Tiziano Vecelli (c. 1488/90–1576) Allegory of Prudence (c. 1565–1570), in a motif redolent of *Janus* in the Introduction. The three heads refer to the three ages of man: youth, maturity and old age. The three-headed animal – dog, lion and wolf – is a symbol of prudence. (Titian, public domain, via Wikimedia Commons.)

The painting portrays three human heads, each facing in a different direction, above three animal heads, from the left, a wolf, a lion and a dog. At the most obvious level of interpretation, the different ages of the three human heads represent the "Three Ages of Man," youth, maturity and old age. Reminiscent of the portrayal of Janus in the Introduction, the different directions in which they are facing reflect the concept of Time itself as having a past, present and future. A third interpretation is suggested by the barely visible inscription "*Ex Praeterito/ Praesens Prudenter Agit/Ne Futura Actione Deturpet*" ("From the experience of the past, the present acts prudently, lest it spoil future actions"). The incorporation of prudence reflected the importance of memory in remembering the past, intelligence to draw lessons in the present and foresight to use these lessons to anticipate wise action in the future.

What of the animal heads, a seemingly bizarre component of the painting? This particular configuration has also been associated with Prudence since Titian's time, and he likely knew that at the time of the painting. Prudence was traditionally depicted as having three heads or faces. The animal head portrayals of a wolf, lion and dog, trace back to a creature that accompanied the Hellenistic Egyptian god Serapis. This three-headed creature was regarded as a metaphor for Time since the 5th century BCE. The voracious wolf represented the past, which devours the memory of all things, the vigorous lion represented the present and the dog represented the future bounding forward.

The painting has been understood in quite a few other ways as well. It has been seen as an allegory about sin and penitence, an admission by Titian that his failure to act prudently in his youth and middle age has condemned him to lead a regretful old age, hence his self-portrayal looking angry, menacing, scowling – and remorseful.

And finally, the lighting of the three faces reveals yet another nuanced interpretation. The aged face is the darkest of the three, with experience and wisdom notwithstanding. It is being eclipsed by the others, with the brightest light of youth being illuminated. This may be Titian's victory statement, an assertion that the prudence that comes with experience and old age is an *essential* aspect of artistic discrimination and judgment, rebutting the notion that old age was the enemy of artistic achievement. The art of any profession is indeed long.

***

An individual's career has a beginning, middle and end. None of these epochs are abrupt but rather a complex choreography and segue from one to the other, constantly building on knowledge, skills and wisdom. *Ars longa, vita brevis.* In a passage of time uncannily congruent with the administration of an anesthetic as well as almost every other aspect of patient care, the fluidity of moving between knowledge, skill and wisdom is both a challenge and a privilege. Like Janus, the past, present and future must guide practice, with a special nod to Hippocrates who valued prognosis as the highest practice of medicine.

The metaphor for the administration of an anesthetic and the practice over a career lifetime also provides insight for guiding one's professional development. It is indeed a matter of time and experience in constantly "monitoring" (just like an anesthetic) optimal interventions for one's own professional future.

The anesthetist watches over the patient in the operating room and him/herself throughout a career of professional and self-development. How those specifics are defined is up to the individual's incorporation of numerous professional values, many of which can be understood within the allegories of personification from so long ago.

INDEX

A
Acedia *214*
Adam, Nicolas-Sébastien *107*
Adikia 166, 235, 242, 243
Aeneas *76*
Aeneid 86
Aergia xiii, 212, 213, 215; *see also* Acedia; Socordia
Aeschylus 15, 34, 159, 166, 167, 185; *Eumenides* 34; Oresteia trilogy 167; *Prometheus Bound* 15; *Seven Against Thebes* 122
Aesop 14–15, 146–47, 171–72
Agamemnon 96, 122, 123, 185
Aglaia 20, 93, 172
Aidos (Aedos) xii, 143, 156–57, 159
Akeso *17*, 20
Akhilles xi, 44, 68, *71–72*, 72, 72–73, 77, *77*, *80*, 185, 200
Akhos *49*, 51
Aldegrever, Heinrich *211*
Aletheia xii, 143, *145*, 146–47
Alexander the Great 56, 123, 229
Algea *49*, 51–52, 116, 236
allegory xiv, xv, xv, 6, 193, 253
altruism 43, 45–46, 178
American Society of Anesthesiologists 26, 43
Amphiareion 35
Anacreonta 51–52
anesthesia: complete reversibility expectation 26, 38, 174; craft, practice of as xiv, 84; early modern history of xv; etymology of xi, 38, 56, 58, 59, 63, 64, 65; hormesis 213–16; "ideal anaesthetic" 26–27; induction, maintenance and emergence 2; as ongoing resuscitation 24; operating procedures 2–3; post-operative visit 3; preoperative consultation 2, 37, 109; public health issues 248; recovery 24–25, 36; "sleep" as proxy for 36, 38; status quo ante 27, 174–75, 213–14; transcendent discomfort of xv, 30; transitions to continuity 175; uncertainty, management of 151; uncertainty and risk 24–25, 29–30, 37–39, 210; varieties of 49–50, 64
Anesthesia Patient Safety Foundation 41–42

256 INDEX

anesthesiologists: as advocates for justice 165, 248–49; boredom and fear 121–22; civic advocacy, training in 248–49; craft and deftness 84; heroic self-image 174; as Janus 3, 5–6; public voice, development of 175; synchronous and asynchronous attention 109–10; uncertainty and fear 45, 46, 109, 122; US personnel xv; wellness of 27
Ania *49*, 51
Anteros 130, 135
Antiphon of Rhamnus 234, 235
Aphrodite: Aeneas and *76*; Aphrodite Urania and Aphrodite Pandemos 92; attributes of 92, 94; beauty and grace of xvi, 91, 92; Cnidus Aphrodite *93*; duality of 92, 94; Erotes and 130, 135, *136*, 137, 138, 172; Harmonia and 117; Hephaistos and 87; Kharites and *114*, 172–73; Pandora and 11; Paris and 117; Phobos and 121, 126
Apollo/Apollon: Apollo Belvedere 94, *95*; Asklepios, father of 18; attributes of 94, 97, 98; beauty and grace of xvi, 94, 98; Dionysus, contrast with 98–99; duality of 94, 96; as healer 23, 98; Hippocratic oath 17–18; as knowledge deity 102; laurel wreath 43; Marsyas and 96–97; Muses and 97; prophecy 97, 104; Syphilis and 12
Apollodorus 18
Arctinus 23
Ares: Anteros and 135; Aphrodite and 93, 95, 117, 122, 134; Athena and 104; Deimos and 123, 124, 134; Enyo and 116–17, 122; Harmonia and 117, 135; Nike and 220; Phobos and 122, 123, 124, 126, 134
Arete *67*, 102, *209*
Aristophanes 130, 131, 187
Aristotle: contemplation 68–69; craft and knowledge 88–89; Eros 130; happiness 178; *Nicomachean Ethics* 178; nomos and physis 235; political animal, man as 228; rhetoric and eloquence 189, 201–03; Theophrastus and 56; truth 148; virtue 160
Artemis 18, 73, 94, 108
Asklepios: asklepian 24; death, blessing of 25; family of xi, *17*, 19–24, 26–27, 96; life of 18–19
assisted suicide 164
Asteria 103, 104, 108
Astraea *163*, 165, 166, 242
Atë 236
Athena: Asklepios and 18; attributes of 103; aulos, invention of 98; birth of 105; Hephaistos and 87; Nike and 219, 221, 225; Pallas and 217; Pandora and 11; Paris and 117; Phobos and Deimos and 126; wisdom 104, 220, *106*

INDEX

Athens: Dark Ages 163; democracy 189, 232, 242–43, 245–47; Hipparchus, death of 232; Hormes, worship of 212; impiety, as crime in 232; Nike, representations of 219; Peloponnesian War 195–96, 227, 234; Pericles' Funeral Oration 195–96; Plague of 227–28; rhetoric and eloquence in 85, 190, 201–02; *School of Athens* (Raphael) *189*; Solon and 168–69, 190, 236, 243; wisdom and cunning, regard for 105
Atropos *29*, 30, 34, 34, *35*, 167
Augustine 186
Avicenna 12, 148

B

beauty and grace: in anesthesiology xvi; burnout as loss of 93; incorporation into daily work 92, 93; medical discourse, neglected in 92; in medical interactions xii, 68, 92; Muses and 86; *see also* Aphrodite; Apollo; Kharites
Beldoch, Michael 118
Bellerophon 44
Beroe 134
Bigelow, Henry Jacob 63
Burne-Jones, Edward *181*

C

Caracci, Annibale *209*, 210
Caravaggio *133*
Cassiodorus 60
Castelli, Pietro 62
Celsus 206–07
Centers for Disease Control and Prevention 164
Chaucer, Geoffrey 87
Chest of Kypselos 38, 166, 242
Christian Church, medical knowledge and 59–60
Cicero 186, *204*, 205
civility ix, xii, 81, 138
Clarke, William xv
collaborative medical practice: civility and xiii; professional voice and xiii; solitary vs. xii, 237–39
Compositiones Medicorum (Scribonius Largus) 58
conscience clauses 164
Consolatio 192, 193–96, 200
consolation: COVID-19 and 193; medical duty to offer 191, 193; neurobiological basis 193–94; professional voice and xiii, 196
Constantinus Africanus 60–61
Coustou, Guillaume, the Younger *83*
COVID-19 pandemic 193, 203–04, 222, 238, 248
craft: of anaesthesia xv–xvi, 84; intellect vs. 87, 102; knowledge, integration with 88–89; *see also* Hephaistos; Muses; Tekhne
Critical Care Medicine 50
cultural competency in health care 164

D

Daniel, Samuel 35
Dante 87

258 INDEX

"De Anaesthesia" (Quistorp) 62–63
De Simplicibus (Galen) 58
deception 149–51; *see also* truth
defeat: clinical mistakes 224; death as medical defeat 222–23; learning from failure 223
Deimos 13, 122, 123–24, 126, 134
democracy: Athenian 190, 232, 242–43, 245–47; demos of health professionals 247–48; elite vs. full enfranchisement 246; etymology of 246–47; rhetoric and 189–90
Demokratia xiii, 247
Demosthenes 243–44, 247–48
Dikaiosyne 165, 167, 243–44
Dike xii, xiii, 143, 165–68, 232, 235, 242–44
Dionysus (Bacchus) 96, 98, 134, 138
Dionysus Soter 42
Dioscorides 55, 57–58, 59, 61
disease: atrophy (*macies*) 13; epilepsy 12; hope and 11, 14–15; as moral punishment 12, *see also* Pandora; plague (*pestis*) 12–13; post-Nomadic emergence of 10; syphilis 11–13; wasting (*tabes*) 13
disruptive physician behavior 184
Donne, John 36
dreams as revelation 34, 36
drugs: Church opposition to 60; ether xv, 63; herbals, classical reliance on 23–24; hyoscyamus 58, 62; loss of knowledge in Dark Ages 58, 60; mandrake/mandragora 55, 56, 57–58, 60, 64, 75; opium 58, 63, 192; Salerno as center of knowledge 61–62
Dysnomia xiii, 235–36

E
effort *see* hormesis
Eliot, Syr Thomas 75
eloquence: basic training 202, 206; considering the audience 203–04; emotional appeal, crucial importance of 201, 202–03; as enhancing acquisition of knowledge 206; in health care xiii, xvi, 201; as public persuasion 201, 203; self-humanization as strategy 202; as Tekhne 84
Epimetheus 11, 14, 108, 109
Epione 19, 25
epistêmê 88, 89, 102
Erasmus 78
Erasistratos 56–57
Eris 45, *113*, 115–17, 122, 146, 235, 237, 243
Eros *129*, *133*; of creation, of philosophers, of erotic poets 130–32; as weapon 132–35; *see also* Aphrodite; Erotes
Eros Farnese 129
Erotes 130, 131, 134, *136*, 134; *see also* Anteros; Eros; Hedylogos; Hermaphroditos 137; Himeros 137–38; Hymenaios 138; Pothos
ether *see* drugs

INDEX

Eudaimonia *114*, 172, 178
Eunomia 185, 235, 235–36, 236, 242, 243, 244
Euripides 156, 157, 168, 185; *Hippolytus* 33, 185
Eusebeia 232, 233
Everett, Edward 63

F
famous artists with medical training 87–88
Fates 34–35, *36*, 166, 167
fear: boredom and 37; fear conditioning 124–25; heroism and 44–45; as impairment to decision-making 45, 123; as intimidation 123, 124; mortality and 45; neurobiology of 124, 125; in operating room xi–xii; patient fear 37; uncertainty and 45, 46, 109, 122
Flexner report 237–38
Foltz, Philipp *194*
Fracastoro, Girolamo 12
Francis (Pope) 168
Frankenstein (Shelley) 108

G
Galen 58, 60
Gawande, Atul 225
Gettysburg Address 196–97
Giambattista della Porta 62
Gilgamesh 4
Goldfarb, Stanley 237
grace *see* beauty and grace
Graces *see* Kharites
Grand Surgery (Guy de Chauliac) 62
Groopman, Jerome 15

Guidelines for the Ethical Practice of Anesthesiology 46
Guy de Chauliac 62

H
Hades 19, 34, 37
Hans von Gersdorff 62
Harmonia *114*, 116, 118, 135, 185
Harmonius and Aristogeiton *231*, 232, 244
harmony in the operating room xi–xii, 114; emotional intelligence 116, 118, 123; empathetic intelligence 118; leadership 118; manipulative emotional intelligence 118; stable teams 115
Hedone 51
Hedylogos 135–36
Heidegger, Martin 168
Hekate 103, 104, 108–09
Hephaistos: Aphrodite and 87, 92, 93, 94; expulsion from Olympos 84; integration of knowledge and craft 88; Kalleis and 92; as knowledge deity 103; Pandora and 10–11; Tekhne and xi, xiv, 68, *83*, 84, 85, 87–88
Herakles 44, 81, 122, 151, *209*, 210
Heraklitus 184–85, 243
Her-ef-ha-ef 4
Hermaphroditos 137
Hermes 11, 98, 137, 219
Herodotus 86, 185
heroism: daring, mortality and fear 44–45; flawed heroes

44; as professional value 45; prosocial 45–46
Hesiod 10–11, 14, 20, 32, 34, 51–52, 85, 106–07, 109, 122, 130, 137, 158, 180, 182–83, 192, 207; *Theogony* 127–28, 141, 193–94; *Works and Days* 138
Hesychia 166
Hilary of Poitiers 59
Himeros 130, 137–38
Hippocrates 56, 58, 60, 62, 98, 109, 179, 182, 193, 206, 253
Hippocratic Collections 53
Hippocratic Oath 17–18, 27, 140
Hitler, Adolf 118
Holmes, Oliver Wendell 56, 63
Homer 30–31, 51, 68, 74–75, 85, 104, 105, 158, 172–73; *Iliad* 23, 30, 98, 99, 116–17, 123–24, 125–26, 167, 182–83, 185, 236–37; *Odyssey* 86, 94, 167, 175, *199*
Homeric Hymns 87
Hope 7, 11–12, 14–15, *181*
Horace 173
Horme and Hormes xiii, 212–13
hormesis 213–16
hubris 69, 159, 160, 173, 184, 186
Hugh of Lucca 61–62
human condition xi, 7, 112, 216
humility 159–60
Hygeia *17*, 19, 23, 24, 25, 27
Hymenaios 138–39
Hypnos 30–32, 38, 213

I
Iapyx *76*
Iaso 20, *21*
implicit bias 165

in vitro fertilization 165
inequality, effects of on patients 164
intellect 103–04
International Association for the Study of Pain 50

J
Janus 3–4, *251*, 252, 253
Jason 44
John of Salisbury 80–81
justice: inequality and 164–65; natural forces, relation to in antiquity 166, 168; obligation to provide medical treatment 164–65; shift from divine to human law 168; social justice 244; varieties of 244; virtue vs. laws and rules 168

K
Kalleis xvi, 92; *see also* Graces
Kalliope xiii, 199–201, 238
Kassirer, Jerome 38
Kharites 51, *91*, 92–93, 137, 172–73, 178, 180
Kheiron: Akhilles and *71*, 72, 73, *77, 80–81*; Asklepios and 18; death of 81–82; dialectic of scholarship and brutality 78–81; as educator of student disciples 72–74, 75–78; as first medical educator 72; pain relief expertise 75; scholarship xi, xiv, 68, 89
Kindler, Albert *181*
kindness: clinical detachment vs. 174–75; compassion, empathy and sympathy

vs. 179; continuity of care 176; effective and efficient in health care 175–76; neurophysiological effects of 178; oikesosis 178; as personal vs. professional value 173; in psychiatry 176; teachability of 176, 178; undermined by increasing medical specialization 177–78; as virtue 173, 176
King, Martin Luther, Jr. 118
Klotho 34
knowledge: augmented by wisdom 102; craft, integration with 88–89; deities of 102–03; *see also* Apollo; Muses
Koios 102–103

L

Lachesis *29*, 30, 34, *36*
Lemoyne, François *152*
Leto 94, 96, 103, 104, 108
Lexicon Medicum Graeco Latinum (Castelli) 62
Liaison Committee on Medical Education 164
Lincoln, Abraham 115, 196–97
Long, Crawford xv
love: all-conquering xii, *133*; collaborative care 137; flattery and 136–37; object yearning and abstract yearning 139; passion for career 138; self-love 137; surgeon and anesthesiologist, metaphorical marriage of 138–39; teacher's love of profession 139–40

Lupe *49*, 51
Lycurgus 220
Lyssa *111*

M

Maccari, Cesare 204
Machai 222
Machiavelli, Niccolò 77–78, 80
Maimonides, prayer of 140
Makhaon 23, 25–26
mandragora *see* drugs
Marsyas 96–97
Materia Medica (Dioscorides) 57–58
Medical Orders for Life-Sustaining Treatment (MOLST) 223
Meditrina 20, *21*, 23
Meidias Painter *114*
Meslamta-ea 4
Metis 102, 105–07
Metsu, Gabriel *241*
Michelangelo *7–8*
Milton, John 87
mindfulness xiv, 3, 46, 102
Minos 134
morality: etymology of 143; interprofessional cooperation and xii; provider–patient relationship xii
Morbidity and Mortality meetings 224
Morpheus 33–34, 213
Morpheus (Restout) *34*
Morton, William T.G. xv, 63, 146
Muses xi, 32, 35, 68, 85–87, 89, 98, 102, 137, *199*; *see also* Kalliope

262   INDEX

Muslim medical knowledge 58–59, 60, 61

N
Nemesis *155*, 156, 159
Nietzsche, Friedrich 99
Nike xiii, *217*, 218–20
Nomos xiii, 232–33
Nonnus of Panopolis 132, 134–35
nous 102
nudity as transparency 25
Nyx xi, *29*, 30, 34, 116, 130, 213; *see also* Fates; Hypnos; Morpheus; Thanatos

O
Odysseus 44
Orpheus 200, 244
Orphic Hymns 19–20
Osler, Sir William 173
Ovid 12, 34, 87, *163*

P
Paean 98
Paidia *114*
pain: Classical distinctions of 51–54; depression and 50, 53–54; gate control theory of 53; metaphysical conception of 52; psychoneuroendocrine response to chronic pain 50; surgical 53–54; as symptom of underlying condition 50; varieties of 50
Palimonies xiii
Palioxis 222
Panakeia 20
Pandora 7, *9*, 10–12, 14, 146, 183

Pandora (Waterhouse) *9*
Pan-Hellenic festivals 229
panic xii
parables xiii
Paracelsus 12, 213
Paregoros xii, 192, 238; *see also* Consolation
patient safety: anaesthesiologists pioneers of 38, 41–42, 43; caution vs. daring intervention xi, 43–44, 46; *primum non nocere* 41–42; *see also* heroism
Pausanias 20, 38, 42–43, 130, 212, 219, 242
Peabody, Francis W. xii, 173
Pericles 190, 194–95
Perseus 44
Persian Wars 229
Philomela 151
Philophrosyne xii, 172–73; *see also* Kharites
Phobos *121*, 122–24, 125, 126
Phoebe 102–03, 108
phrenes 182–83
phronesis 102
pimping 89
Pindar 19, 86, 92, 138, 146, 173, 232, 235
Pistis 146
Plato: doctors 177; *Charmides* 185; *Crito* 234–35, 245; Eros and Erotes 130, 138–39; justice 237, 242–43; nomos and physis 235; *Protagoras* 243; *Republic* 185, 186–87, 237; requited love 135; sophrosyne 185, 186–87; soul, location of 182; truth 148
Pliny the Elder 74

Plutarch 123
Podaleirios 23, 25
polis: justice in 237, 242–45; nomos vs. physis 233–35; as social form 228–29
Polycraticus (John of Salisbury) 80–81
Porphyry 178
Pothos 138
Poussin, Nicolas *1–2*
Practica Chirurgiae (Roger Frugardi) 61–62
pragmatism 102
Praxiteles *95*
prelapsarian myths 7
Procne 151
professional coaching in medicine 224–25
professionalism: definition, difficulty of xiii; emotions, importance of mastering 112; enduring qualities necessary for 68–69; enriching anemic conceptions of xiii, xv; etymology of ix–xi; formal benchmarks vs. professional growth 72; life phases of a career 253–54; operating room as crucible for ix, 114; "staying in one's own lane" vs. social engagement 237–39
prognostication 53, 98, 104, 105, 108–10, 253
Prometheus 10–12, 81, 102–03, 106–09, 146–47
prophecy: Apollo 97–98; Hekate 108; Koios 103; Phoebe 108; Themis 165; *see also* prognostication
prosocial actions 45–47
prosopopoeia 193
prudence *251*, 252–53
Pseudo-Apuleius 59
Pseudologoi 146–47

Q

Quistorp, J.B. 62–63

R

Raphael *189*
Reagan, Ronald 195–96
respect: for patients 156; for trainees 156; self-respect 159, 160; shame and 157, 159
restitution vs. quest narrative of medical care 174–75
Restout, Jean-Bernard *34*
rhetoric *see Consolatio*; eloquence
Richmond, Julius 27
Roger Frugardi 61
Romulus 4
Rosa, Salvator *163*

S

Sabine women 4
safety *see* patient safety
Salerno 61–62
Sappho 138
scholarship xi, 68
Scott, Walter 34
Scribonius Largus 58
Seneca 52–53
Seneca the Younger 192
Serapis 252
Sertürner, Friedrich 33
Shakespeare, William 87; *Hamlet* 37, 125, 156–57; *Othello* 3, 5

shame: anxiety and 158–59; guilt vs. 157–58; humility and 159–60; as moral motivator 158, 160–61; respect and 156–57, 159
Shelley, Mary 108
Simonides 232
skill xi, 68
Socordia *211*, 212
Socratic teaching 89
Solon 86, 168, 190, 236, 243
Sophia xi, xiv, 68, *101*
Sophocles 168, 185; *Antigone* 233
Sophrosyne xii, *181*, 182–183, 184–86
Soteria *41*, 42
Sparta 123, 185
Stoics 178, 186
strife in the operating room: "blood-brain barrier" xii; conflict resolution training 115; detrimental to patient care 114–15; positive aspects of 115–16; surgeons and 114–15
support networks for physicians 225
Sweerts, Michiel *227*
systems theory 115
Szent-Györgyi, Albert 99

T
Tekhne xi, xiv, 68, 84, 88, 89
Telesphoros 23, 25
Temperantia (Burne-Jones) *181*
Tereus 151
Thanatos 31, 32–33, 37, 38, 213
Themis *144*, 165, 167, 242
Theodoric of Cervia 61–62

Theophrastus 56, 57
Theseus 44
Thomas Aquinas 148, 186
Thrasymachus 243–244
Thucydides 185, 228, 234
Titian *251*, 252–53
Trojan War 23, 42, 44, 73, 75, 96, 117
truth: coherence theory 149; consensus theory 149; constructivist theory 149; correspondence theory 149; honesty and 147; integrity 148; time and 151–52; transparency and 148; *see also* deception
Turner, William 62

U
Unequal Treatment (Institute of Medicine report) 164
Updike, John 82
Urania *199*
Usmu 4

V
Vergerius, Petrus Paulus 205
Veritas *see* Aletheia
victory as conquest over disease 222, 225
Virgil 13, 86
voice, professional xiii, xv, 84–85, 238
Vouet, Simon *199*

W
Warren, John Collins xv
Waterhouse, John William *9*
wellness, concept of 26, 27, 98
wisdom: knowledge, augmented by wisdom 102;

nous and epistêmê 102; phronesis, pragmatism and mindfulness 102; as ultimate professional step xi, 68; *see also* Athena; Metis

Z

Zeus: Asclepius and 19, 96; Bellerophon and 44; deceit of 151; Dike and 166, 242, 243, 244; Hephaistos and 87; Hypnos and 30; Metis and 105–6; Nike and 217–18, 219, *221*, 225; Nomos and 232; Pandora and 10–11, 14; Pothos and 138; Prometheus and 106–108; Titans and 103–04; Typhoeus and 132, 134

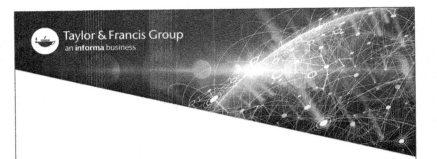